KU-362-533

Evidence-based Cardiology

Second edition

Volume I

Provided as a service to medical education by

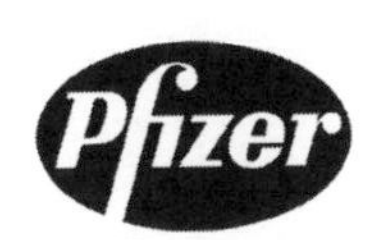

Evidence-based Cardiology

Second edition

Volume I

Edited by

Salim Yusuf
Heart and Stroke Foundation of Ontario Research Chair, Senior Scientist of the Canadian Institute of Health Research Director of Cardiology and Professor of Medicine, McMaster University, Hamilton Health Sciences, Hamilton, Canada

John A Cairns
Dean, Faculty of Medicine, University of British Columbia, Vancouver, Canada

A John Camm
Professor of Clinical Cardiology and Chief, Department of Cardiological Sciences, St George's Hospital Medical School, London, UK

Ernest L Fallen
Professor Emeritus, McMaster University, Faculty of Health Sciences, Hamilton, Canada

Bernard J Gersh
Consultant in Cardiovascular Diseases and Internal Medicine, Mayo Clinic; Professor of Medicine, Mayo Medical School, Rochester, Minnesota, USA

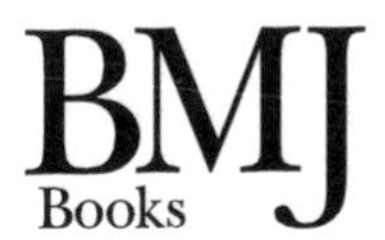

BMJ Books is an imprint of the BMJ Publishing Group

Second edition first published in 2003
First edition published in 1998
Second impression 1999
by BMJ Books, BMA House, Tavistock Square,
London WC1H 9JR

www.bmjbooks.com

British Library Cataloguing in Publication Data
A catalogue record for this book is available from the British Library

ISBN 0 7279 1704 8

Typeset by Newgen Imaging Systems (P) Ltd.
Printed and bound by MPG Books, Bodmin, Cornwall

Contents

Contributors vii
Preface to the Second edition ix
Preface to the First edition xi
Glossary xiii

Part I: General concepts and critical appraisal **1**
Salim Yusuf, Editor

1 What is evidence-based cardiology? 3
PJ Devereaux, R Brian Haynes, Salim Yusuf

2 A critical appraisal of the cardiovascular history and physical examination 14
Akbar Panju, Brenda Hemmelgarn, Jim Nishikawa, Deborah Cook, Allan Kitching

3 Obtaining incremental information from diagnostic tests 23
Raymond J Gibbons

4 Clinical trials and meta-analysis 34
Colin Baigent

5 Finding current best evidence to practice evidence-based cardiology 40
Dereck L Hunt, K Ann McKibbon, R Brian Haynes

6 Understanding concepts related to health economics 46
Mark Hlatky

7 Introduction to decision analysis 56
Kevin A Schulman, Henry A Glick, Allan S Detsky

8 Assessing and changing cardiovascular clinical practices 71
C David Naylor, David A Alter

Index 89

Contributors

David A Alter
Institute for Clinical Evaluation Sciences
Deparment of Medicine
University of Toronto
Toronto, Canada

Colin Baigent
Clinical Trial Service Unit and Epidemiological Studies Unit
University of Oxford
Oxford, UK

Deborah Cook
Professor, Department of Medicine
McMaster University
Hamilton, Canada

Allan S Detsky
Departments of Health Administration and Medicine
University of Toronto
Toronto, Canada

PJ Devereaux
Department of Medicine
McMaster University
Hamilton, Canada

Raymond J Gibbons
Nuclear Cardiology Laboratory
Mayo Medical School
Mayo Clinic
Rochester, USA

Henry A Glick
Assistant Professor
University of Pennsylvania School of Medicine
Philadelphia, Pennsylvania, USA

R Brian Haynes
Health Information Research Unit
Department of Clinical Epidemiology and Biostatistics
McMaster University Faculty of Health Sciences
Hamilton, Canada

Brenda Hemmelgarn
Nephrology, Department of Medicine
University of Calgary
Calgary, Alberta, Canada

Mark Hlatky
Department of Health Research and Policy
Department of Medicine
Stanford University School of Medicine
Stanford CA, USA

Dereck L Hunt
Department of Clinical Epidemiology and Biostatistics
McMaster University
Hamilton, Canada

Allan Kitching
Assistant Clinical Professor
Department of Medicine
McMaster University
Hamilton, Canada

K Ann McKibbon
Health Information Research Unit
McMaster University
Hamilton, Canada

C David Naylor
Sunnybrook HSC
University of Toronto
Toronto, Canada

Jim Nishikawa
Associate Professor
Department of Medicine
University of Ottawa
Ottawa, Ontario, Canada

Akbar Panju
Professor, Department of Medicine
McMaster University
Chief, Department of Medicine
Hamilton Health Sciences
Hamilton, Canada

Kevin A Schulman
Center for Clinical and Genetic Economics
Duke Clinical Research Institute
Duke University Medical Center
Durham, USA

Preface to the Second edition

"Where is the knowledge in all that information?
Where is the wisdom in all that knowledge?"
W H Auden

The recent proliferation of carefully controlled large scale clinical trials, their meta-analyses and selective observational studies has contributed to the remarkable strides made in the management of cardiovascular disease. One of the prophesies stated in the first edition of this textbook has come to pass – namely, that management guided by external evidence is an evolving process as newer and more effective treatment modalities come to light. While successful as a critical approach for managing patients, evidence-based medicine is nevertheless a work in progress which, if allowed to rest on its laurels, will "by nature be threatened with impending obsolescence". In addition to keeping abreast of new information, there is a need to integrate and distill the information into coherent recommendations. Authors were therefore instructed to provide their recommendations including those based on qualitative judgments. The recognition of new developments in a rapidly changing dynamic field combined with the overwhelmingly positive worldwide response to the first edition have prompted the publication of this second edition.

This edition is again dedicated to providing a comprehensive compendium of best evidence for the diagnosis and management of a wide variety of cardiovascular disorders. To avoid critical information gaps as meaningful new data emerge, the text contains several new features. Because our concepts of what constitutes evidence-based medicine is subject to change we have included a completely revised introductory chapter. Appended to the printed text is a CD Rom that permits ready access to new information and periodic updates by way of a dedicated and active website. In addition, there will be available a compact hand-held (PDA) version of the text. There are new chapters on clinical trials and meta-analysis; fetal origins of cardiovascular disease; genetics; diet and cardiovascular disease; obesity; and cardiopulmonary resuscitation. Several chapters have been completely rewritten and most have undergone substantial revision. Finally, the layout of the text has been reformatted for better handling, portability, readability and affordability.

In preparing this edition the editors and contributors have subscribed to the principle that the best external evidence found in these pages are not to be considered as hierarchical choices but rather should be used judiciously with other forms of evidence be they pathophysiologic, observational or experiential. No effort has been spared in the preparation of this edition and to this end invaluable assistance has been accorded us by Judy Lindeman at McMaster University and Mary Banks and Christina Karaviotis at BMJ Books.

Salim Yusuf
John A Cairns
A John Camm
Ernest L Fallen
Bernard J Gersh

Preface to the First edition

> "... if a man declares to you that he has found facts that he has observed and confirmed with his own experience, be cautious in accepting what he says. Rather, investigate and weigh this opinion or hypothesis according to requirements of pure logic, without paying attention to this contention that he affirms empirically."
>
> MOSES MAIMONIDES. *ca.* 1195

Thus did the great physician Maimonides make a plea for an evidence-based approach to medicine by admonishing his followers to seek common ground between objectivism and empiricism. If Maimonides had lived in the year 1785, he would likely have read William Withering's *An Account of the Foxglove*; a compendium of Withering's personal observations on the clinical effect of the digitalis leaf. At first blush, Maimonides would cry foul at such flagrant empiricism, demanding to know the whole of the inception cohort. It turns out that Withering, instead of selecting specific cases which would have "... spoken strong in favour of the medicine, and perhaps been flattering to my own reputation" went on to say in his Preface "I have therefore mentioned every case in which I have prescribed the foxglove, proper or improper, successful or otherwise ..." thus heralding a genuine, albeit retrospective, cohort study. It took 212 years before Withering was ultimately vindicated by the results of the first large scale randomized placebo controlled trial of digoxin (*N Engl J Med* 1997; **336**: 526). Sixty-eight hundred patients with congestive heart failure, in sinus rhythm, were randomized to receive digoxin (avg dose 0·25 mg/day) or placebo in addition to ACE inhibitors and diuretics. Over a three-year period there was no statistical difference in overall mortality but digoxin proved to be effective in reducing hospitalizations due to worsening heart failure.

The advent of large scale prospective randomized clinical trials has strengthened the external evidence upon which management decisions can be made with some confidence. We have come to rely on so-called external best evidence as critical guideposts for establishing minimal criteria for treatment of many cardiovascular disorders. In the process, some myths based on putative mechanisms have been dispelled while insights into the efficacy of new treatments have been more rapidly facilitated. On the other hand there is a danger of righteous complacency which, if unchecked, could lead to a slavish dependency on statistical bottom lines and, ultimately, to "cook book" medicine. It is the intent of this textbook to present a proper balance between "objectivism and empiricism". In this regard, the very first chapter begins by defining the practice of evidence-based cardiology as "... integrating individual clinical expertise with the best available external clinical evidence from systematic research".

The textbook has four principal components. An introductory general section addresses important topics in clinical epidemiology, as applied both to the bedside and to a population. This section includes: critical appraisal of data; clinical trials methodology; quality of life measurements; health economics; and methods of decision analysis, all in the context of current clinical practice. Next follows a section on preventive strategies based on evidence that should enable the practicing physician to advise, with confidence, on risk factor modification and quality of life issues for selected patients. There follows a section on a broad range of specific cardiovascular disorders that highlight management issues based on current best evidence. Finally, the section on clinical applications is an attempt to put a clinical face on evidence derived from population statistics through the use of "live" clinical cases. Here, an attempt is made judiciously to couple external evidence with clinical expertise and a sound knowledge of cardiovascular pathophysiology. There is understandably a wide range of the kinds of evidence available to support different practices and treatments. The editors have chosen not to constrain the authors into rigid and uniform formats for each chapter. While several of the chapters have the level of evidence/recommendations graded, or key messages highlighted, a uniform format would not have been appropriate for every chapter.

This textbook is designed for a wide audience. Since cardiovascular disease comprises more than fifty percent of adult medicine, there is something here for everyone in clinical practice and at all levels of medical undergraduate and postgraduate training. Its emphasis on practical applications of research methodology and critical appraisal of data covering a cross-section of clinical topics should invite interest among those engaged in population studies, biostatistics, clinical epidemiology and health economics as well as those involved in healthcare decision analysis, quality assurance committees and stakeholders responsible for healthcare planning.

Because this textbook relies so heavily on current best evidence, it is by nature threatened with impending obsolescence. To ensure that this does not happen, the editors, in concert with the publisher, have agreed to issue up-dates periodically in the form of special supplements or updated editions, so that the text can be continually revised in accordance with emerging relevant data. In this context, it is well to bear in mind that good science always proceeds hesitantly through a series of tenuous conclusions. And so any recommendation made on the basis of available best evidence is subject to revision as we probe deeper into the mysterious nature of disease processes. One may ask of the large scale clinical trial "Why did it require more than 10,000 patients to show incontrovertible evidence that the experimental drug is effective?" Aye, there is the scientific question!

The editors wish to acknowledge the herculean efforts of Catherine Wright and Karin Dearness who kept everyone on track and offer a special appreciation to Mary Banks for her editorial expertise, patience and support.

Salim Yusuf
John A Cairns
A John Camm
Ernest L Fallen
Bernard J Gersh

Glossary

Abbreviations commonly used in this book

ABI	ankle brachial pressure index
ACC	American College of Cardiology
ACE	angiotensin-converting enzyme
AED	automated external defibrillator
AF	atrial fibrillation
AHA	American Heart Association
AMI	acute myocardial infarction
APSAC	anisoylated plasminogen streptokinase activator complex
APTT	activated partial thromboplastin time
ARR	associated risk reduction
AS	aortic stenosis
ASD	atrial septal defect
ASMR	age standardized mortality rate
BBB	bundle branch block
BMI	body mass index
CABG	coronary artery bypass grafting
CAD	coronary artery disease
CBVD	cerebrovascular disease
CCB	calcium-channel blockers
CCU	coronary care unit
CEE	conjugated equine estrogen
CHD	coronary heart disease
CHF	congestive heart failure
CI	confidence interval
CK-MB	creatinine kinase MB isoenzyme
CPP	coronary perfusion pressure
CPR	cardiopulmonary resuscitation
CT	computerized tomography
CYA	cyclophosphamide
DA	dopamine
DALY	disability adjusted life years
DHP	dihydropyridines
DM	diabetes mellitus
DVT	deep vein thrombosis
ECG	electrocardiogram
EEG	electroencephalogram
EGF	epidermal growth factor
EMF	endomyocardial fibrosis
EOA	effective orifice area
EPS	electrophysiologic studies
FGF	fibroblast growth factor
FS	fractional shortening
GPI	glycoprotein inhibitor
HCM	hypertrophic cardiomyopathy
HDL	high density lipoprotein (HDL_2)
HMG-CoA	3-hydroxy-3-methylglutaryl-coenzyme A
HOCM	hypertrophic obstructive cardiomyopathy
HRT	hormone replacement therapy
IC	intracoronary
ICD	implantable cardioverter defibrillator
ICH	intracerebral hemorrhage
IDC	idiopathic dilated cardiomyopathy
IDL	intermediate density lipoprotein
IE	infective endocarditis
IFN-γ	interferon gamma
IGF	insulin-like growth factor
IGT	impaired glucose tolerance
IL	interleukin
IM	intramuscular
INR	international normalization ratio
IQR	interquartile range
IV	intravenous
LAE	left atrial enlargement
LBBB	left bundle branch block
LDL	low density lipoprotein
LDL-C	low density lipoprotein cholesterol
LMWH	low molecular weight heparin
Lp(a)	lipoprotein
LQTS	long QT syndrome
LV	left ventricular
LVE	left ventricular enlargement
LVEF	left ventricular ejection fraction
LVH	left ventricular hypertrophy
MCP	monocyte chemoattractant protein
MHC	major histocompatibility complex
MHS	Milan Hypertensive Strain
MI	myocardial infarction
MPA	medroxyprogesterone acetate
MRI	magnetic resonance imaging
MUFA	monounsaturated fatty acid
NA	not available
NHLBI	National Heart Lung Blood Institute
NINDS	National Institute of Neurologic Disease and Stroke
NNT	number needed to treat
NSAIDs	non-steroidal anti-inflammatory drugs
NSTEMI	non-ST-segment elevation myocardial infarction
NYHA	New York Heart Association
OR	odds ratio
P	probability
PAI	plasminogen activator inhibitor
PCI	percutaneous coronary intervention
PCR	polymerase chain reaction
PDGF	platelet derived growth factor
PE	pulmonary embolism
PET	positron emission tomography
PPCM	peripartum cardiomyopathy
PSVT	paroxysmal supraventricular tachycardia
PTA	percutaneous transluminal angioplasty
PTCA	percutaneous transluminal coronary angioplasty

PUFA	polyunsaturated fatty acid
PVC	premature ventricular complex
RCT	randomized controlled trial
RFLP	restriction fragment length polymorphisms
ROSC	return of spontaneous circulation
RRR	relative risk reduction
rtPA	recombinant tissue plasminogen activator
RV	right ventricular
RVEF	right ventricular ejection fraction
RVF	right ventricular enlargement
RVH	right ventricular hypertrophy
SAECG	signal-averaged ECG
SC	subcutaneous
SK	streptokinase
SMC	smooth muscle cells
SFA	saturated fatty acid
SFA	superficial femoral artery
STEMI	ST-segment elevation myocardial infarction
TEA	thromboendarterectomy
TEE	transesophageal echocardiography
t-FA	*trans* fatty acid
TGF	transforming growth factor
TIA	transient ischemic attack
TIMI	Thrombolysis in Myocardial Infarction
TMP	TIMI myocardial perfusion
TNF	tumor necrosis factor
TNK	tenecteplase
tPA	tissue plasminogen activator
TTE	transthoracic echocardiography
UK	urokinase
v	versus
VF	ventricular fibrillation
VPD	ventricular premature depolarization
VSD	ventricular septal defect
VT	ventricular tachycardia
VTE	venous thromboembolism
VUI	venous ultrasound imaging

Grading of recommendations and levels of evidence used in *Evidence-based Cardiology*

GRADE A

Level 1a Evidence from large randomized clinical trials (RCTs) or systematic reviews (including meta-analyses) of multiple randomized trials which collectively has at least as much data as one single well-defined trial.

Level 1b Evidence from at least one "All or None" high quality cohort study; in which ALL patients died/failed with conventional therapy and some survived/succeeded with the new therapy (for example, chemotherapy for tuberculosis, meningitis, or defibrillation for ventricular fibrillation); or in which many died/failed with conventional therapy and NONE died/failed with the new therapy (for example, penicillin for pneumococcal infections).

Level 1c Evidence from at least one moderate-sized RCT or a meta-analysis of small trials which collectively only has a moderate number of patients.

Level 1d Evidence from at least one RCT.

GRADE B

Level 2 Evidence from at least one high quality study of nonrandomized cohorts who did and did not receive the new therapy.

Level 3 Evidence from at least one high quality case–control study.

Level 4 Evidence from at least one high quality case series.

GRADE C

Level 5 Opinions from experts without reference or access to any of the foregoing (for example, argument from physiology, bench research or first principles).

A comprehensive approach would incorporate many different types of evidence (for example, RCTs, non-RCTs, epidemiologic studies, and experimental data), and examine the architecture of the information for consistency, coherence and clarity. Occasionally the evidence does not completely fit into neat compartments. For example, there may not be an RCT that demonstrates a reduction in mortality in individuals with stable angina with the use of β blockers, but there is overwhelming evidence that mortality is reduced following MI. In such cases, some may recommend use of β blockers in angina patients with the expectation that some extrapolation from post-MI trials is warranted. This could be expressed as Grade A/C. In other instances (for example, smoking cessation or a pacemaker for complete heart block), the non-randomized data are so overwhelmingly clear and biologically plausible that it would be reasonable to consider these interventions as Grade A.

Recommendation grades appear either within the text, for example, **Grade A** and **Grade A1a** or within a table in the chapter.

The grading system clearly is only applicable to preventive or therapeutic interventions. It is not applicable to many other types of data such as descriptive, genetic or pathophysiologic.

Part I

General concepts and critical appraisal

Salim Yusuf, Editor

Grading of recommendations and levels of evidence used in *Evidence-based Cardiology*

GRADE A

Level 1a Evidence from large randomized clinical trials (RCTs) or systematic reviews (including meta-analyses) of multiple randomized trials which collectively has at least as much data as one single well-defined trial.

Level 1b Evidence from at least one "All or None" high quality cohort study; in which ALL patients died/failed with conventional therapy and some survived/succeeded with the new therapy (for example, chemotherapy for tuberculosis, meningitis, or defibrillation for ventricular fibrillation); or in which many died/failed with conventional therapy and NONE died/failed with the new therapy (for example, penicillin for pneumococcal infections).

Level 1c Evidence from at least one moderate-sized RCT or a meta-analysis of small trials which collectively only has a moderate number of patients.

Level 1d Evidence from at least one RCT.

GRADE B

Level 2 Evidence from at least one high quality study of non-randomized cohorts who did and did not receive the new therapy.

Level 3 Evidence from at least one high quality case–control study.

Level 4 Evidence from at least one high quality case series.

GRADE C

Level 5 Opinions from experts without reference or access to any of the foregoing (for example, argument from physiology, bench research or first principles).

A comprehensive approach would incorporate many different types of evidence (for example, RCTs, non-RCTs, epidemiologic studies, and experimental data), and examine the architecture of the information for consistency, coherence and clarity. Occasionally the evidence does not completely fit into neat compartments. For example, there may not be an RCT that demonstrates a reduction in mortality in individuals with stable angina with the use of β blockers, but there is overwhelming evidence that mortality is reduced following MI. In such cases, some may recommend use of β blockers in angina patients with the expectation that some extrapolation from post-MI trials is warranted. This could be expressed as Grade A/C. In other instances (for example, smoking cessation or a pacemaker for complete heart block), the non-randomized data are so overwhelmingly clear and biologically plausible that it would be reasonable to consider these interventions as Grade A.

Recommendation grades appear either within the text, for example, **Grade A** and **Grade A1a** or within a table in the chapter.

The grading system clearly is only applicable to preventive or therapeutic interventions. It is not applicable to many other types of data such as descriptive, genetic or pathophysiologic.

1 What is evidence-based cardiology?

PJ Devereaux, R Brian Haynes, Salim Yusuf

Introduction

In 1836 the editor of the *American Journal of Medical Sciences*, Elisha Bartlett, heralded a study as "one of the most important medical works of the present century, marking the start of a new era in science".[1] What evoked such praise and suggested a paradigm shift was Dr Pierre Louis' systematic collection and numerical presentation of data on bloodletting. Louis adopted a baconian approach of collecting vast amounts of data on a large number of patients (by the standards of the early 1800s), which allowed him to systematically evaluate the efficacy of bloodletting. Louis argued that large numbers of patients and enumeration were necessary to equalize differences between treatment groups, as "by so doing, the errors (which are inevitable), being the same in two groups of patients subjected to different treatment, mutually compensate each other, and they may be disregarded without sensibly affecting the exactness of the results".[2] Louis subsequently went on to state: "a therapeutic agent cannot be employed with any discrimination or probability of success in a given case, unless its general efficacy, in analogous cases, has been previously ascertained", and thus, "without the aid of statistics nothing like real medicine is possible".[3]

The prevailing concept of illness at the time was that the sick were contaminated, whether by some toxin or contagion, or by an excess of one humour or another. This understanding of illness contained within it the idea that these states were improved by opening a vein and letting the sickness run out. Louis' finding that bloodletting hastened the death of the ill was a bombshell. George Washington had 2·4 liters of blood drained from him in the 15 hours prior to his death: he had been suffering from a fever, sore throat and respiratory difficulties for 24 hours.[4] Some have stated that in this way Washington was murdered.[5–7]

Although this is a relatively recent example, the plea for comparative evaluation was mentioned as early as the Old Testament. Throughout history there have been repeated exhortations to quantify medical or health problems and to compare outcomes in patient groups managed differently, with the goal of setting state policy or assisting individual physicians.

In this chapter we will discuss what evidence-based medicine is, and then discuss an approach to evidence-based decision making. We will use a clinical case to highlight the components of this approach, which include clinical state and circumstances, patients' preferences and actions, research evidence, and clinical expertise. At the end of the chapter we will review the application of these components of evidence-based decision making as they apply to our patient, and provide a decision aid that can be used in such a case.

What is evidence-based medicine?

Although the foundations for evidence-based medicine were laid over several centuries, an explicit philosophy, with its attendant concepts, definitions and models, has been largely developed as a formal doctrine over the last few decades. Evidence-based medicine is about solving clinical problems. Initially, the focus of evidence-based medicine was largely to find the best objective quantifiable research evidence relevant to the particular problem, and to apply that evidence in resolving the particular issue.[8] This early focus de-emphasized "intuition, unsystematic clinical experience, and pathophysiologic rationale as sufficient grounds for clinical decision making" and stressed "the examination of evidence from clinical research".[9] Subsequent versions have emphasized that research evidence alone is never sufficient to make a clinical decision.[10] Research evidence by itself rarely tells us what to do in individual situations, but rather it provides useful information that allows us to make more informed decisions. Clinicians must always view evidence in the context of the individual patient, and then weigh the potential benefits versus the risks, costs and inconveniences. Ideally the patient's values and preferences take precedence[10] (Figure 1.1).

Figure 1.1 is based on the first edition of *Evidence-based medicine*[11] and was published in an editorial that appeared in *ACP Journal Club* and *Evidence-Based Medicine* in 1996, along with the definition: "Evidence-based medicine is the conscientious and judicious use of current best evidence from clinical care research in the management of individual patients".[12] The editorial also included the caveat that the definition of evidence-based medicine would evolve as new types of information emerged, and would therefore be continuously refined. The concepts of evidence-based

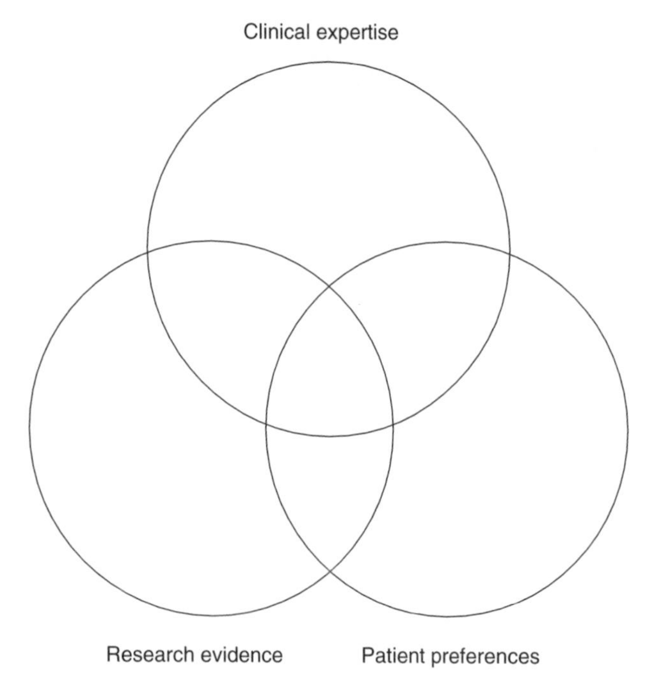

Figure 1.1 Early model of the key elements for evidence-based clinical decisions

medicine have evolved considerably and the initial model has recently been enhanced,[8] especially for what is meant by clinical expertise and the additional consideration of clinical situation and circumstances. In the next section we use this new model of "evidence-based clinical decisions" to help resolve a common clinical scenario.

Approach to evidence-based clinical decision making

New model for evidence-based clinical decisions (Figure 1.2)

Figure 1.2 depicts the evolution of the model for evidence-based clinical decisions,[8] which has more recently been redefined as "the integration of best research evidence with clinical expertise and patient values".[13] This model represents a desirable approach as to how all clinical decisions should be made. However, we acknowledge that, at present, many clinical decisions are not made in this way. For instance, at present, clinicians' individual preferences (as distinct from clinical expertise) often play a large role in their actions, leading to large "practice variations" in managing similar cases. When faced with critically ill patients with identical circumstances, different clinicians may, according to their preferences, institute aggressive life-prolonging interventions or withdraw life support.[14] Our model acknowledges that patients' preferences should be considered first and foremost, rather than clinicians' preferences, whenever it is possible to do so.

In Figure 1.2, the "clinical state and circumstances" of the patient replace "clinical expertise" as one of the key elements in clinical decisions, "patient preferences" is expanded to include patients' actions, and this element is reversed in position with "research evidence", signifying its frequent precedence. Integrating all three aspects requires judgment and clinical expertise, thus constituting a fourth overarching element. We will describe each of the components, and the role of clinical expertise in integrating them.

Clinical state and circumstances

A patient's clinical state and circumstances often play a dominant role in clinical decisions. Clinical trials provide us with results reflective of the average patient within the treatment groups of the trial, but rarely is a patient in

Clinical scenario

A family physician refers a patient requesting your input on the issue of antithrombotic therapy. The patient is an 80 year old man with a history of hypertension who 10 months ago, on routine examination, was diagnosed with atrial fibrillation. The patient suffered a major gastrointestinal bleed, requiring hospitalization, urgent endoscopy, and a transfusion the day after his atrial fibrillation was discovered (the patient had not started any antithrombotic therapy prior to his bleeding episode). He had, however, been receiving a non-steroidal anti-inflammatory drug (NSAID) for osteoarthritis. The patient has been free of any gastrointestinal symptoms since his bleed and has successfully avoided using an NSAID by using acetaminophen. Eight months earlier the patient's echocardiogram demonstrated normal valvular and left ventricular function and a left atrial measurement of 6·5 cm. Based on the duration of atrial fibrillation and the size of his left atrium, you decide that cardioversion is not an option. The patient is very worried about having a stroke, as his wife was left dependent on him for 2 years prior to her death following a major stroke. The referring physician, who recently had a patient who suffered a serious gastrointestinal bleed while on warfarin, is very concerned about the risk of bleeding, given this patient's age and recent history of gastrointestinal bleeding.

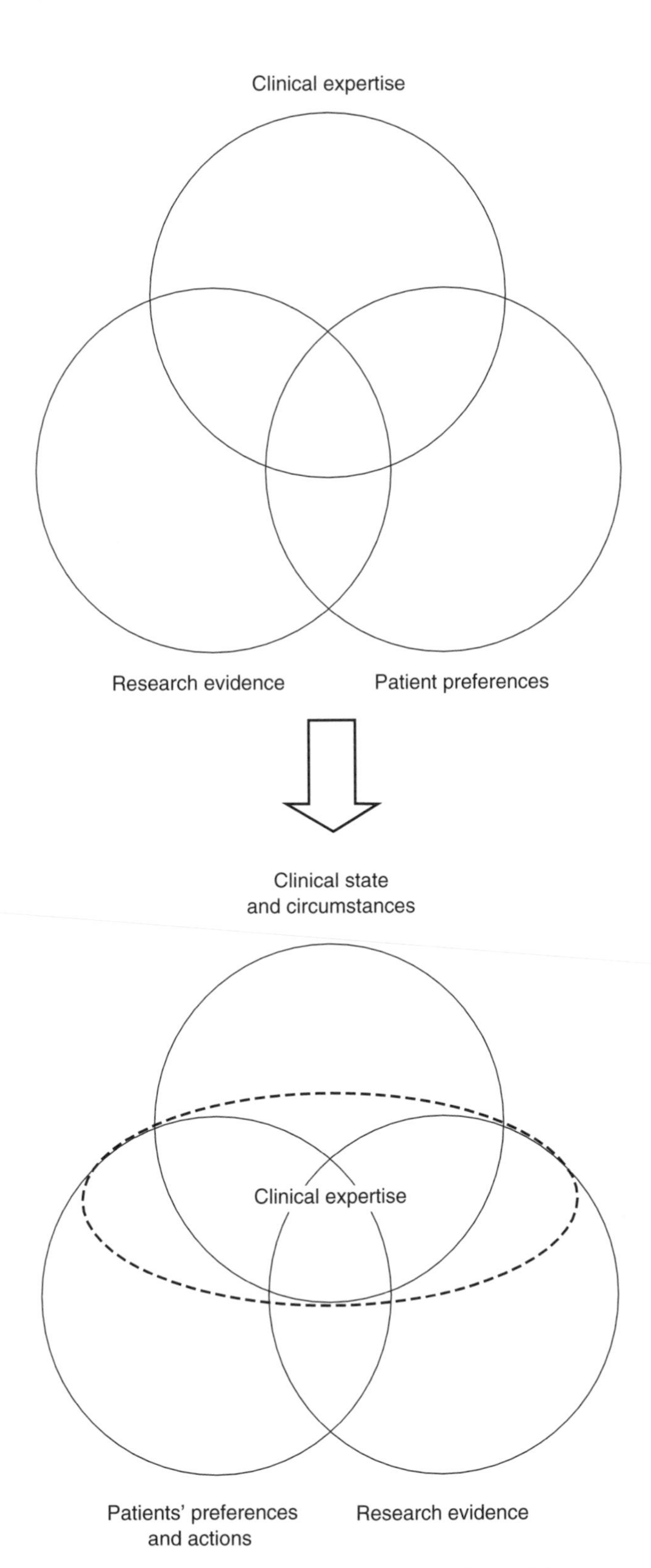

Figure 1.2 Evolving model for evidence-based clinical decisions

clinical practice the same as the average patient from a clinical trial. Individual patients have unique characteristics that typically put them at lower or higher risk of the outcome or treatment side effect than the average patient in the trial. As such, optimal clinical decisions should be individualized to the patient's clinical state. A patient who is at very high risk of a future vascular event, but at low risk of any complication from a drug (for example, a patient with a low density lipoprotein value of 8·0 mmol/l post myocardial infarction and no contraindication to statin therapy), or conversely a patient who is at low risk of the outcome and high risk of a treatment's complications (for example, a 40 year old man with atrial fibrillation without any associated stroke risk factors who has experienced a recent major gastrointestinal bleed), may find their clinical state dominating the clinical decision making process.

It is notable that the circles of clinical state and circumstances and research evidence overlap. Frequently research evidence can inform us about the influence of the clinical state and circumstances. Considering our patient, the pooled data from five randomized controlled trials (RCTs) evaluating the efficacy of warfarin in patients with non-valvular atrial fibrillation (NVAF) demonstrated an average annual stroke rate of 4·5% and a major bleeding rate of 1% in patients not receiving antithrombotic therapy.[15] The investigators who combined the five RCTs used the control patient data to develop a clinical prediction tool to estimate the annual risk of stroke. Independent risk factors that predicted stroke in control patients were increasing age, a history of hypertension, diabetes, and prior stroke or transient ischemic attack (TIA).[15] Our patient's annual risk of stroke is predicted to be about 8%, which is higher than that of the average control patient in the five RCTs, whose annual stroke rate was 4·5%.[15] Similarly, a clinical prediction tool has been developed for predicting the risk of major bleeding (defined as the loss of two units of blood within 7 days, or life-threatening bleeding) while taking warfarin therapy.[16] Independent risk factors that predict major bleeding in patients taking warfarin include age >65, history of stroke, history of gastrointestinal bleeding, recent myocardial infarction, anemia, renal failure and diabetes. (Note that many of the factors that predict a higher risk of stroke also increase the risk of bleeding.) Our patient's annual risk of major bleeding of 8% also differs from that of the average patient receiving warfarin in the five RCTs, whose annual risk of major bleeding was 1·3%. We are unaware of any clinical prediction tool for predicting major bleeding while taking aspirin, and the atrial fibrillation trials had inadequate power to estimate this. However, based on the results of the meta-analysis by the antithrombotic trialists' collaboration, we would expect aspirin to increase the risk of major bleeding from 1% to about 1·3% on average.[17]

The clinical circumstances in which you and your patient find yourselves (for example, your ability to administer and monitor a treatment) may be very different from those of an RCT. For example, the patient may not be able to obtain frequent tests of the intensity of anticoagulation. However, for a patient with the same clinical characteristics, we can frequently optimize clinical circumstances to decrease the risk of an outcome or treatment side effect. For example, we can decrease the risk of bleeding due to warfarin therapy by more intensive monitoring. Thus, an "evidence-based" decision about anticoagulation for a patient with atrial fibrillation is not only determined by the demonstrated efficacy of anticoagulation and its potential adverse effects,[18] but will vary based on the patient's clinical state and according to individual clinical circumstances.

Patients' preferences and actions

Patients may have no views or, alternatively, unshakable views, on their treatment options, depending on their condition, personal values and experiences, degree of aversion to risk, healthcare insurance and resources, family, willingness to take medicines, accurate or misleading information at hand, and so on.[8] Accordingly, individuals with very similar clinical states and circumstances may choose very different courses of action, despite being presented with the same information about the benefits and risks of an intervention.

For our patient with NVAF, research evidence informs us about the differing preferences of patients and their physicians for antithrombotic therapy in atrial fibrillation when they weigh the competing risks of stroke and bleeding.[19] In this study,[19] participants (that is both physicians and patients) reviewed flip charts describing in detail the acute and long-term consequences of a major and minor stroke and a major bleeding event. Participants were instructed that the likelihood of a minor or major stroke was equal. The participants then underwent a probability trade-off technique which determined the minimum number of strokes that needed to be prevented before the participant felt antithrombotic therapy was justified (this value was determined for both warfarin and aspirin), given the associated increased risk of bleeding, costs and inconveniences. The same technique was also used to determine the maximum number of excess bleeds the participant would consider to be acceptable with antithrombotic therapy (determined both for warfarin and aspirin), given the benefits in terms of stroke reduction with this therapy. This study demonstrates significant variability between physicians and patients in their weighing of the potential outcomes associated with atrial fibrillation and its treatment. Patients required less stroke reduction and were more tolerant of the risk of bleeding than physicians. For example, on average, patients were willing to accept the risk of 17 extra major bleeding events in 100 patients over a 2 year period if warfarin prevented eight strokes among these 100 patients. Physicians, however, were only willing to accept 10 major bleeding events for the same level of benefit. Furthermore, physicians varied significantly in how much bleeding risk they thought was acceptable for a given stroke reduction associated with an antithrombotic agent. Hence different physicians would make very different recommendations to the same patient with identical risks of bleeding and stroke. This underscores the importance of having patient values and preferences drive clinical decision making. It is the patient who is at risk of the outcome and so, when willing and able, they should be the one to weigh the potential benefits versus the risks, costs and inconveniences.

There is debate regarding the optimal way to elicit and incorporate patient preferences into clinical decision making. One method is to discuss the potential benefits and risks with a patient and then qualitatively incorporate your impression of the patient's preferences into the clinical decision. Alternatively, at least two quantitative approaches exist: decision analytic modeling and probability trade-off technique. In a decision analytic model, a standard gamble, time trade-off or visual analog scale technique is used to determine the utility (patient value/preference) of the various outcomes. This information is then fed into a decision tree that includes the probabilities of the outcomes for all clinical decisions being considered. Using the decision tree, calculations are undertaken to determine what course of action optimally fits the patient's preferences. The probability trade-off technique presents patients with the probabilities for the various interventions being considered and then asks them to make a decision based on this information. This allows a direct and quantitative incorporation of the patient's preferences.

Proponents of decision analytic modeling question whether patients can understand probabilities to allow the appropriate incorporation of their preferences. Proponents of probability trade-off techniques wonder if a measure of utility (that is preference) in the absence of probabilities is meaningful. Only one study has directly compared decision analytic modeling with a probability trade-off technique.[20] This study focused on the primary prevention of stroke and myocardial infarction with aspirin therapy in elderly patients. Both methods (that is decision analysis and probability trade-off) were performed on all patients at separate times. This study demonstrated that treatment recommendations varied significantly, depending on which method was used. After patients were presented with their individual treatment thresholds as determined by both methods, over twice as many stated they would base their preferences on the results of the probability trade-off as opposed to the decision analysis.[20] Further research is needed to determine which of the models better represents patients' self-interests.

Regardless of what their preferences may be, patients' actions may differ from both their preferences and their clinicians' advice.[21] For example, a patient may prefer to lose weight, quit smoking and take their medications as prescribed, but their actions may fall short of achieving any of these objectives. Alternatively, they may follow the treatment as prescribed, even if they resent its imposition, adverse effects and costs. Unfortunately, clinicians' estimates of their patients' adherence to prescribed treatments have no better than chance accuracy.[22] Thus, physicians' decisions for care will better meet the model's specifications if they are able to assess whether their patients will follow, or are following, their prescriptions.[22]

We recognize that at present patients' preferences are rarely formally incorporated in clinical practice. This may be related to lack of physician training in these approaches, a reluctance to tread unfamiliar ground, and also in many circumstances the lack of accurate quantitative information on risk and benefits, as well as clinical risk prediction tools. However, this is likely to change rapidly as clinical models can be derived from large databases and handheld computers can be utilized to quantify risks and benefits at the bedside.

Research evidence

We support a very broad definition of research evidence, namely, "any empirical observation about the apparent relation between events".[23] In keeping with this definition, research evidence includes everything from the unsystematic observation of a single physician to a systematic review of large RCTs. Not all evidence is created equal, and hence there is a hierarchy of evidence that varies depending on whether one is addressing a diagnostic, prognostic or therapeutic decision. We will focus on the hierarchy of evidence for therapeutic decisions (Box 1.1).[23]

Box 1.1 Hierarchy of evidence for treatment decisions*

Coherence of evidence from multiple sources
Systematic review of several well designed, large randomized controlled trials
Single large randomized controlled trial
Systematic review of several well designed small randomized controlled trials
Single small randomized controlled trial
Systematic review of several well designed observational studies
Single observational study
Physiologic studies
Unsystematic observation from a physician

* This hierarchy cannot be rigidly adhered to. At times a single observation may be very powerful (for example, defibrillation for ventricular fibrillation), or observational studies may provide unequivocal evidence (for example, smoking cessation and lung cancer). However, in most cases where treatment effects may be moderate, outcomes variable or the clinical course unpredictable, the proposed hierarchy is useful.

All evidence has value, and the best evidence available in the hierarchy should be given appropriate consideration, even if not at the top of the hierarchy. Therefore, the unsystematic observations of colleagues should not be dismissed when no higher level evidence exists. Indeed, unsystematic observations can lead to many important insights, and experienced clinicians usually develop a respect for the insights of their astute colleagues. However, it is equally important to recognize that unsystematic observations are commonly limited by the small number of observations, variability in outcomes, lack of objectivity, and the difficulties in integrating (for example, taking into account the natural history of a disorder, placebo effect, and a patient's desire to please) and drawing inferences from observations.[24]

All evidence has limitations. Although the majority of advances in medicine are initially uncovered through individual observations, physiologic studies, observational studies or randomized controlled trials evaluating surrogate endpoints, there have also been several extremely misleading findings that have, at times, resulted in harm. It is important to remember that contradictory results across studies on the hierarchy of evidence table are not isolated to one or two instances (Table 1.1).

Perhaps the most powerful example is the story of antiarrhythmic therapy. Despite encouraging evidence that encainide and flecainide could prevent premature ventricular beats, a large RCT demonstrated a higher mortality rate with these drugs than with placebo, such that these drugs resulted in an extra death for every 20 patients treated with encainide or Flecainide.[39] It is estimated that more Americans were killed by these drugs than died in the Vietnam War.[40]

Ideally, we would have evidence from all levels of the hierarchy and the evidence would be coherent across all levels. This would represent the most persuasive evidence. However, this rarely happens, as even RCTs may by chance frequently demonstrate contradictory findings, especially when they are small. Therefore, physicians should always aim for the highest level of evidence for clinical decision making. Clinicians can still make strong inferences, particularly when there is evidence from a systematic review of several well designed large RCTs, or simply a large single pragmatic RCT. The RCT is such a powerful tool because randomization is our only means to reduce bias in treatment comparisons by controlling for unknown prognostic factors.[41] Therefore, RCTs have the potential to provide the most valid (that is likelihood that the trial results are unbiased) estimates of treatment effect.[42] Furthermore, large RCTs with broad eligibility criteria enhance the generalizability of their findings.

An *n* of 1 randomized controlled trial is an RCT where individual patients are randomized to pairs of treatment periods, such that they receive the experimental treatment during one period and a placebo during the other.[43] Both patients and healthcare providers are blind to which period is the experimental and which the placebo. Patients continue undergoing pairs of treatment periods until they and the healthcare providers become convinced that the experimental intervention either does or does not work.[43] The advantage of an *n* of 1 RCT is that it provides evidence directly from the patient. However, this method is applicable only in a disease state that has limited fluctuation, and

Table 1.1 Some examples of contradictory results across studies at various positions in the hierarchy of evidence

Results from lower level evidence	Results from higher level evidence
Milrinone demonstrated improvement in left ventricular function during exercise[25]	A large RCT[26] and meta-analysis of several RCTs[27] demonstrated a 28% relative increase in mortality with milrinone compared to placebo
An observational study of extracranial to intracranial bypass surgery suggested a "dramatic improvement in the symptomatology of virtually all patients" undergoing the procedure[28]	A large RCT demonstrated a 14% relative increase in the risk of fatal and non-fatal stroke in patients undergoing this procedure compared to medical management[29]
A meta-analysis of 16 cohort studies and 3 cross-sectional angiographic studies (including studies of women with known coronary artery disease) demonstrated a relative risk of 0·5 (95% CI 0·44–0·57) for coronary artery disease among women taking estrogen[30]	A moderate-sized secondary prevention RCT did not demonstrate any reduction in coronary heart disease events but did demonstrate an increase in thromboembolic events in patients receiving estrogen.[31] Preliminary reports from an ongoing very large RCT (Women's Health Initiative) indicate an increased risk of MI and strokes in the first 2 years of estrogen therapy[32]
A secondary analysis of an RCT suggested that lower doses of ASA were associated with a higher risk of perioperative stroke and death in patients undergoing carotid endarterectomy[33]	A large prospective RCT showed a higher risk of perioperative stroke, myocardial infarction or death with high-dose ASA[33]
A physiologic study demonstrated that β blockers result in a decline in ejection fraction and increases in end-diastolic volume in patients with prior myocardial infarction[34]	A meta-analysis of 18 RCTs[35] and 3 large trials (CIBIS–2,[36] MERIT-HF[37] and COPERNICUS[38]) in patients with heart failure found a 32% relative risk reduction in death in patients receiving β blockers

for treatments that can be crossed over (for example, short-acting medical treatments rather than surgery) and which are targeted at symptom relief and quality of life, as opposed to serious outcomes such as myocardial infarction and death. Even then, *n* of 1 RCTs are not feasible for many patients because of lack of infrastructure to support them, such as a pharmacy that is able and willing to provide matching placebos. Also, short-term symptomatic effects of treatments may differ from their long-term effects, so that *n* of 1 trials may provide misleading answers. Similarly, if side effects occur only after prolonged treatment (for example, during to drug accumulation, as with amiodarone), then short-term crossover studies (which is what *n* of 1 trials are) may not identify the full risks associated with a treatment. As such, there has been limited implementation of *n* of 1 RCTs in cardiology, but they represent a unique opportunity (when possible and applicable) to obtain individual patient level evidence.

Considering our case of the patient with NVAF, the highest level of evidence comes from a systematic review of all the RCTs that have evaluated antithrombotic therapy in patients with atrial fibrillation.[18] This study demonstrates that warfarin reduces the relative of stroke (ischemic and hemorrhagic) by 62%, and aspirin by 22%.

Considering the risk of bleeding associated with warfarin therapy, there is an RCT that demonstrates a 50% decrease in the risk of bleeding if a patient is willing to undergo education, training and self-monitoring of prothrombin time.[44]

Clinical expertise

Evidence-based decision making requires clinical expertise to establish and balance the patient's clinical state and circumstances, preferences and actions, and the best research evidence. Before a therapeutic decision can be considered, clinical expertise is required to get the diagnosis and prognosis right. As shown above, clinical prediction tools can be extremely helpful in determining a patient's prognosis, but they are unlikely to eliminate the need for sound clinical judgment acquired through clinical experience. Sizing up the clinical circumstances has never been more challenging, as commonly there exist several potential interventions, some of which require technical expertise for their effective and safe delivery. Getting the evidence right requires the skill to identify, evaluate and apply the evidence appropriately. Communicating with patients has always been considered important. This takes on greater importance as there is a growing desire on the part of patients to be involved in decisions relating to their health. Expertise is required to provide patients with the information they need, to elicit their preferences, and to incorporate those preferences into the decision.

Currently there is no consensus on how this information should be presented to patients and how their preferences should be incorporated. However, we know that information should not be presented in relative terms (for example, warfarin will decrease your risk of stroke by 62%) because patients assume their baseline risk is 100% even when they are instructed it is not.[45] A recent systematic review of RCTs that compared decision aids (that is interventions designed to help people make specific choices among options by providing information on those options and outcomes relevant to the patient's health) to traditional ways of involving/informing patients in decision making[46] demonstrated that decision aids, as opposed to usual care, improved the average knowledge scores of patients for the options and outcomes by 20% (95% CI 13–25), reduced decisional conflict scores (that is patients felt more certain, informed, and clear about values in their decision), and increased patient participation in decision making.[46] Where available, decision aids provide a potential means to facilitate information presentation, incorporation of preferences, and participation in the decision-making process.

The varying roles of the components of evidence-based clinical decisions

Depending on the circumstances, any of the circles in the new model could predominate. Varying the size of the circles to reflect their actual contribution to the clinical decision could portray this visually. Sometimes the clinical state or circumstance dominates the clinical decision. For example, a patient who is at very high risk of an outcome and low risk of a complication may have their clinical state dominate the decision-making process. A patient living in a remote area may not have access to anticoagulation monitoring, and this would probably dominate the decision-making process. Patient's preferences can be so strong that they act as the driving factor in the decision-making process. For example, some patients will not take blood products regardless of the clinical situation. Research evidence can be the main factor in decision making when the benefit of an intervention is moderate to large in size and the risk of treatment small, as with β blocker therapy in patients post myocardial infarction, ACE inhibitors in coronary artery disease or heart failure, or cholesterol lowering with statins. Finally, clinical expertise can predominate, especially when it is related to technical capabilities.

Application to our patient

For our patient the evidence would suggest an 8% annual risk of stroke and 1% risk of major bleeding without any antithrombotic therapy. With warfarin therapy we would expect the annual risk of stroke to decrease to 3% and the risk of major bleeding to increase to 8%. This latter could be reduced to 4% if the patient were willing to undergo self-monitoring of their prothrombin time and an education program, as discussed above.[44] With aspirin therapy we would expect the annual risk of stroke to decrease to 6% and the risk of major bleeding to increase to 1·3%.

As discussed above, there is no consensus on how to present this information to our patient or how to incorporate his preferences. We have provided a decision aid for patients that describes atrial fibrillation (Table 1.2), a major and minor stroke (Table 1.3), a severe bleed (Table 1.4), and a probability trade-off for no treatment, aspirin and warfarin therapies (Figure 1.3). The descriptions of major and minor stroke and a severe bleed are slight modifications of the descriptions developed and tested by Man-Son-Hing and colleagues.[47] We have also individualized the probability trade-off for our patient, with the knowledge that he would undergo self-monitoring of his prothrombin time if he decided to take warfarin therapy (Figure 1.4).

Once this evidence-based clinical decision is reached our job is not over. The patient will need monitoring to ensure he is able to follow through on his clinical decision. One advantage of the decision aid provided (including his individualized probability trade-off) is that the patient can take the information home and does not have to rely on his memory to recall the facts discussed during your meeting.

Table 1.2 Atrial fibrillation: the most common disorder of the heartbeat

Risk	Chances of developing atrial fibrillation increase with age and it occurs in approximately 10% of all people above the age of 75
Physical symptoms	Irregular and usually rapid beating of the heart, sensed as a fluttering in the chest. Some patients feel no symptoms and are unaware that they have atrial fibrillation
Complications	Stroke • Atrial fibrillation increases the risk of a clot developing in the heart. This clot can be swept up towards the brain, causing a stroke • The chance of developing a stroke with atrial fibrillation increases with either age greater than 65 years, high blood pressure, diabetes, heart failure, or a history of strokes or "mini-strokes" • The risk of developing a stroke with atrial fibrillation varies, depending on how many of these risk factors you have
Treatment	• There are medications that thin the blood, which help to prevent clots and therefore stroke • Because the blood is thinned there is an increased risk of bleeding

Table 1.3 ☹ Strokes ☹ can be minor or major in severity. If you have a stroke as a result of atrial fibrillation, your chance of having a minor or major stroke are equal

	Minor stroke	Major stroke
Physical symptoms	You suddenly cannot move or feel one arm and one leg	You suddenly are unable to move one arm and one leg You cannot swallow
Mental symptoms	You are unable to fully understand what is being said to you You have difficulty expressing yourself	You are unable to understand what is being said You are unable to speak
Pain	You feel no physical pain	You feel no physical pain
Recovery	You are admitted to hospital Your weakness, numbness and problem with understanding improve, but you still feel slightly weak or numb in one arm and one leg You are able to do almost all of the activities you did before the stroke You can function independently You leave the hospital after 1 week	You are admitted to hospital You cannot dress The nurses feed you You cannot walk After 1 month of physiotherapy you are able to wiggle your toes and lift your arm off the bed You remain this way for the rest of your life
Further risk	You have an increased risk of having more strokes	Another illness will probably cause your death

Table 1.4 ☹ Severe ☹ bleeding while taking warfarin or ASA: an example of a stomach bleed

Physical	You feel unwell for 2 days, then suddenly you vomit blood
Treatment	You are admitted to hospital You stop taking warfarin or ASA A doctor puts a tube down your throat to see where you are bleeding from You receive sedation to ease the discomfort of the test You do not need an operation You receive blood transfusions to replace the blood you lost
Recovery	You stay in hospital for 1 week You feel well at the end of your hospital stay You need to take pills for the next 6 months to prevent further bleeding After that you are back to normal

Bleeding from the stomach is the most common type of serious bleeding while taking warfarin or ASA; however, rarely other serious forms of bleeding can occur, such as bleeding within the head after a fall.
Warfarin or ASA can also cause minor bleeding, including bruising and nose bleeds.
Taking warfarin can mean costs and inconvenience to yourself and family. For example: need for blood tests; parking/transportation; cost of warfarin.
Taking ASA can mean costs to yourself.
For example: cost of ASA.

Limitations of evidence-based clinical decision model

This model does not consider the important roles that society, governments or healthcare organizations can play in decision making. We deliberately restricted ourselves to decisions made by patients and their healthcare providers to allow a focused exploration of the issues involved in their immediate decision making process. However, a healthcare organization may pre-empt these decisions. For example, not funding primary percutaneous transluminal coronary angioplasty in acute myocardial infarction can have an enormous impact on health outcomes, and will impose a clinical decision on all patients and physicians by eliminating this option. Physicians will have to factor in such issues when considering their patient's clinical circumstances.

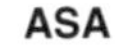

Without any blood thinning medication
Chance of stroke over next 2 years
is _____ out of 100
Chance of severe bleeding over next 2 years
is _____ out of 100

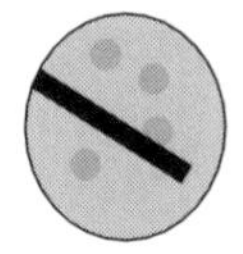

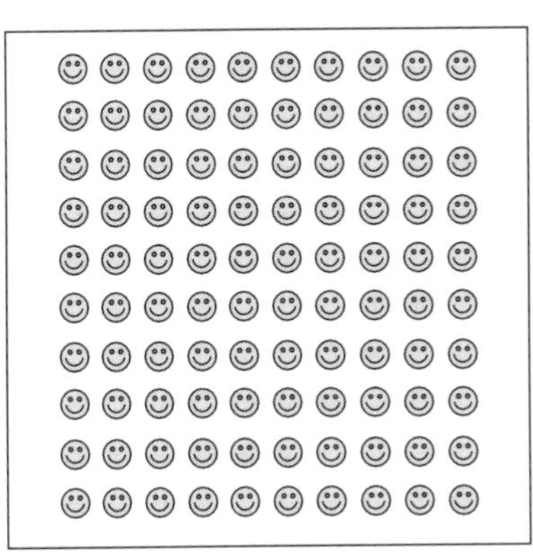

ASA
Chance of stroke over next 2 years
is _____ out of 100
Chance of severe bleeding over next 2 years
is _____ out of 100

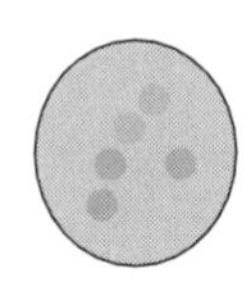

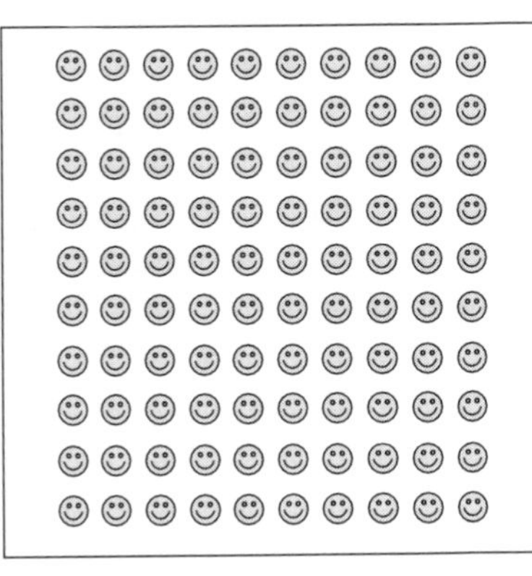

Warfarin
Chance of stroke over next 2 years
is _____ out of 100
Chance of severe bleeding over next 2 years
is _____ out of 100

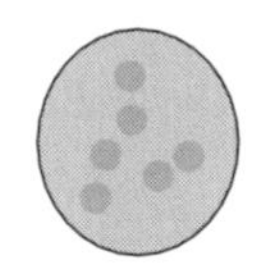

Figure 1.3

Without any blood thinning medication
Chance of stroke over next 2 years
is __8__ out of 100
Chance of severe bleeding over next 2 years
is __1__ out of 100

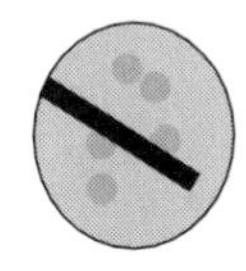

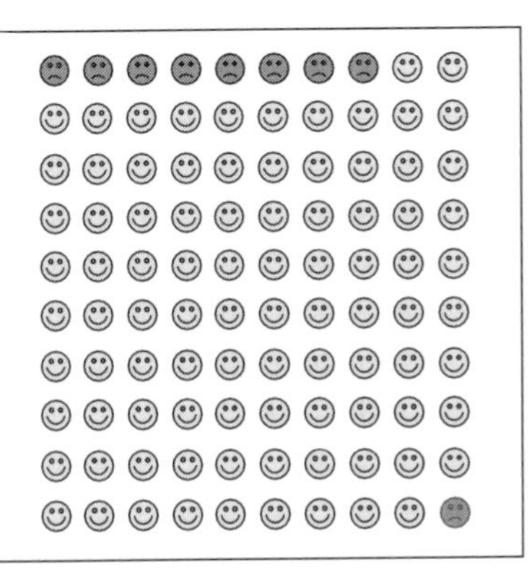

ASA
Chance of stroke over next 2 years
is __6__ out of 100
Chance of severe bleeding over next 2 years
is __1·3__ out of 100 (i.e.13 out of 1000)

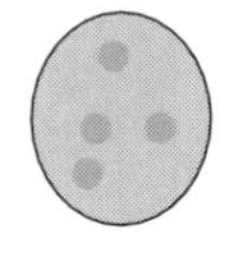

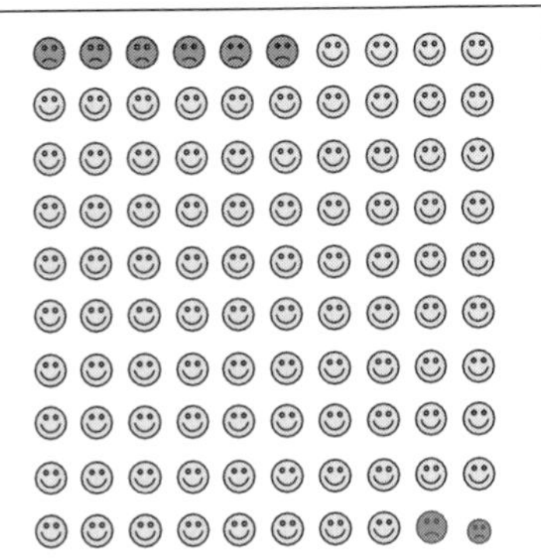

Warfarin
Chance of stroke over next 2 years
is __3__ out of 100
Chance of severe bleeding over next 2 years
is __4__ out of 100

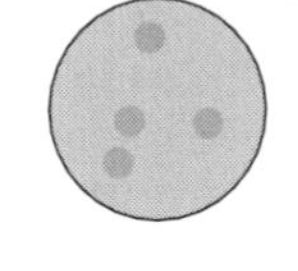

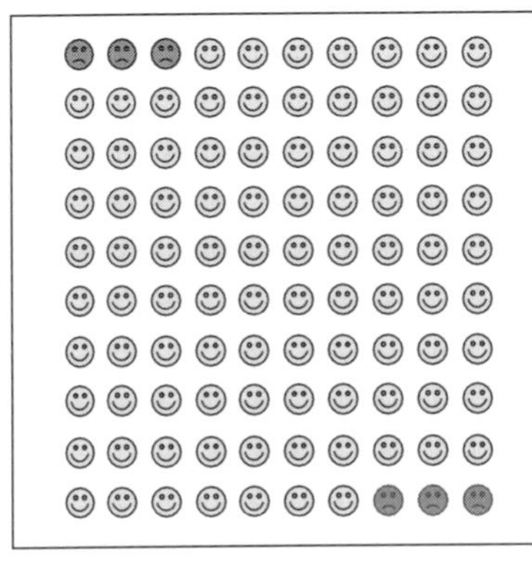

Figure 1.4

Conclusions

The foundations for evidence-based medicine have been established over the centuries but the specific philosophies, concepts, definitions and models have essentially evolved over the past few decades. Evidence-based medicine is about solving clinical problems. Evidence-based decision making depends upon utilizing clinical expertise to integrate information about a patient's clinical setting and circumstances with the best research evidence while incorporating the patient's preferences and actions.

References

1. Louis PCA. Researches on the effects of blood-letting in some inflammatory diseases, and on the influence of tartarised antimony and vesication in pneumonitis. *Am J Med Sci* 1836;**18**:102–11.
2. Louis PCA. *Researches on the Effects of Bloodletting in Some Inflammatory Diseases and on the Influence of Tartarised Antimony and Vesication in Pneumonitis.* Translated by CG Putnam. Boston: Hilliard, Gray, 1836.
3. Louis PCA. Medical statistics. *Am J Med Sci* 1837;**21**:525–8.
4. Morens DM. Death of a president. *N Engl J Med* 1999;**341**:1845–9.
5. Lloyd JU. Who killed George Washington? *Eclectic Med J* 1923;**83**:353–6, 403–8, 453–6.
6. Marx R. A medical profile of George Washington. *Am Heritage* 1955;**6**:43–7, 106–7.
7. Pirrucello F. How the doctors killed George Washington. *Chicago Tribune Magazine* 20 February 1977.
8. Haynes RB, Devereaux PJ, Guyatt GH. Clinical expertise in the era of evidence-based medicine and patient choice. *ACP Journal Club* 2002;**136**:A11–A13.
9. Evidence-based medicine working group. Evidence-based medicine, a new approach to teaching the practice of medicine. *JAMA* 1992;**268**:2420–5.
10. Haynes RB, Sackett DL, Gray JMA, Cook DC, Guyatt GH. Transferring evidence from research into practice: 1. The role of clinical care research evidence in clinical decisions. *ACP Journal Club* 1996;**125**:A-14. *Evidence-Based Medicine* 1996;**1**:196.
11. Sackett DL, Richardson SR, Rosenberg W, Haynes RB. *Evidence-Based Medicine: how to practice and teach EBM.* London: Churchill Livingstone, 1997.
12. Sackett DL, Rosenberg WMC, Gray JA, Haynes RB, Richardson WS. Evidence-Based Medicine: What it is and what it isn't. *BMJ* 1996;**312**:71–2.
13. Sackett DL, Straus S, Richardson SR, Rosenberg W, Haynes RB. *Evidence-Based Medicine: how to practice and teach EBM,* 2nd edn. London: Churchill Livingstone, 2000.
14. Cook DJ, Guyatt GH, Jaeschke R. Determinants in Canadian health care workers of the decision to withdraw life support from the critically ill. *JAMA* 1995;**273**:703–8.
15. Atrial Fibrillation Investigators. Risk factors for stroke and efficacy of antithrombotic therapy in atrial fibrillation. *Arch Intern Med* 1994;**154**:1449–57.
16. Beyth RJ, Quinn LM, Landefeld S. Prospective evaluation of an index for predicting the risk of major bleeding in outpatients treated with warfarin. *Am J Med* 1998;**105**:91–9.
17. Antithrombotic Trialists' Collaboration. Collaborative meta-analysis of randomised trials of antiplatelet therapy for prevention of death, myocardial infarction, and stroke in high risk patients. *BMJ* 2002;**324**:71–86.
18. Hart RG, Benavente O, McBride R, Pearce LA. Antithrombotic therapy to prevent stroke in patients with atrial fibrillation: a meta-analysis. *Ann Intern Med* 1999;**131**: 492–501.
19. Devereaux PJ, Anderson DR, Gardner MJ *et al.* Differences between perspectives of physicians and patients on anticoagulation in patients with atrial fibrillation: observational study. *BMJ* 2001;**323**:1218–22.
20. Man-Son-Hing M, Laupacis A, O'Connor AM, Coyle D, Berquist R, McAlister F. Patient preference-based treatment thresholds and recommendations: a comparison of decision-analytic modeling with the probability-tradeoff technique. *Med Decis Making* 2000;**20**:394–403.
21. Haynes RB. Improving patient adherence: State of the art, with a special focus on medication taking for cardiovascular disorders. In: Burke LE, Okene IS, eds. *Patient Compliance in Healthcare and Research.* American Heart Association Monograph Series. Armonk, NY: Futura Publishing Co, 2001.
22. Stephenson BJ, Rowe BH, Macharia WM, Leon G, Haynes RB. Is this patient taking their medication? *JAMA* 1993; **269**:2779–81.
23. Guyatt G, Haynes B, Jaeschke R *et al.* Introduction: the philosophy of evidence-based medicine. In: Guyatt G, Rennie DR, eds. *Users' guides to the medical literature.* AMA Press, 2002.
24. Nisbett R, Ross L. *Human Inference.* Englewood Cliffs, NJ: Prentice-Hall, 1980.
25. Timmis AD, Smyth P, Jewith DE. Milrinone in heart failure: effects on exercise haemodynamics during short term treatment. *Br Heart J* 1985;**54**:42–7.
26. Packer M, Carver JR, Rodeheffer RJ *et al.* Effect of oral milrinone on mortality in severe chronic heart failure. The PROMISE Study Research Group. *N Engl J Med* 1991; **325**:1468–75.
27. Yusuf S, Teo KK. Inotropic agents increase mortality in patients with congestive heart failure. American Heart Association 63rd Scientific Sessions. Dallas (Texas), 12–15 November 1990. *Circulation* 1990;**82**(SIII):673.
28. Popp AJ, Chater N. Extracranial to intracranial vascular anastomosis for occlusive cerebrovascular disease: experience in 110 patients. *Surgery* 1977;**82**:648–54.
29. Failure of extracranial–intracranial arterial bypass to reduce the risk of ischemic stroke: results of an international randomized trial. The EC/IC Bypass Study Group. *N Engl J Med* 1985;**313**:1191–200.
30. Stampfer MJ, Colditz GA. Estrogen replacement therapy and coronary heart disease: a quantitative assessment of the epidemiologic evidence. *Prev Med* 1991;**20**:47–63.
31. Hulley S, Grady D, Bush T *et al.* Randomized trial of estrogen plus progestin for secondary prevention of coronary artery disease in postmenopausal women. Heart and Estrogen/progestin Replacement Study (HERS) Research Group. *JAMA* 1998;**280**:605–13.
32. http://www.nhlbi.nih.gov/whi/hrt.htm

33.Taylor DW, Barnett HJ, Haynes RB *et al.* Low-dose and high-dose acetylsalicylic acid for patients undergoing carotid endarterectomy: a randomised controlled trial. ASA and Carotid Endarterectomy (ACE) Trial Collaborators. *Lancet* 1999;**353**:2179–84.
34.Coltart J, Alderman EL, Robison SC, Harrison DC. Effect of propranolol on left ventricular function, segmental wall motion, and diastolic pressure-volume relation in man. *Br Heart J* 1975;**37**:357–64.
35.Lechat P, Packer M, Chalon S, Cucherat M, Arab T, Boissel JP. Clinical effects of beta-adrenergic blockade in chronic heart failure: a meta-analysis of double-blind, placebo-controlled, randomized trials. *Circulation* 1998;**98**:1184–91.
36.CIBIS-II Investigators and Committees. The Cardiac Insufficiency Bisoprolol Study II (CIBIS-II): a randomised trial. *Lancet* 1999;**353**:9–13.
37.The MERIT-HF Study Group. Effect of metoprolol CR/XL in chronic heart failure: Metoprolol CR/XL Randomised Intervention Trial in Congestive Heart Failure (MERIT-HF). *Lancet* 1999;**353**:2001–7.
38.Packer M, Coats AJ, Fowler MB *et al.* Effect of carvedilol on survival in severe chronic heart failure. *N Engl J Med* 2001;**344**:1651–8.
39.Echt DS, Liebson PR, Mitchell LB. Mortality and morbidity in patients receiving encainide, flecainide, or placebo: The Cardiac Arrhythmia Suppression Trial. *N Engl J Med* 1991; **324**:781–8.
40.Moore TJ. Excess mortality estimates. *Deadly medicine: why tens of thousands of heart patients died in America's worst drug disaster.* New York: Simon & Schuster, 1995.
41.Kunz R, Oxman AD. The unpredictability paradox: review of empirical comparisons of randomised and non-randomised clinical trials. *BMJ* 1998;**317**:1185–90.
42.Chalmers I. Unbiased, relevant, and reliable assessments in health care. *BMJ* 1998;**317**:1167–8.
43.Guyatt GH, Sackett DL, Taylor DW *et al.* Determining optimal therapy: randomized trials in individual patients. *N Engl J Med* 1986;**314**:889–92.
44.Beyth RJ, Quinn L, Landefeld CS. A multicomponent intervention to prevent major bleeding complications in older patients receiving warfarin. *Ann Intern Med* 2000; **133**:687–95.
45.Malenka DJ, Baron JA, Johansen S, Wahrenberger JW, Ross JM. The framing effect of relative and absolute risk. *J Gen Intern Med* 1993;**8**:543–8.
46.O'Connor AM, Rostom A, Fiset V *et al.* Decision aids for patients facing health treatment or screening decisions: a systematic review. *BMJ* 1999;**319**:731–4.
47.Man-Son-Hing M, Laupacis A, O'Connor A *et al.* Warfarin for atrial fibrillation: The patient's perspective. *Arch Intern Med* 1996;**156**:1841–8.

2 A critical appraisal of the cardiovascular history and physical examination

Akbar Panju, Brenda Hemmelgarn, Jim Nishikawa, Deborah Cook, Allan Kitching

There have been numerous technological advances made in the diagnosis and treatment of cardiovascular disease. In spite of this, a carefully conducted clinical examination remains the cornerstone in the initial assessment of the patient with known or suspected cardiovascular disease. Before conducting further laboratory or radiologic diagnostic tests, clinicians implicitly consider each piece of historical information and each finding from the physical examination as a diagnostic test that increases or decreases the probability of the possible diagnoses. The competency and accuracy of the clinical examination is therefore crucial, for it serves as the basis for our judgment regarding not only diagnosis, but prognosis and therapy as well.

This chapter is not intended to provide details of how to perform a cardiovascular history and physical examination, and should be read in conjunction with standard textbooks on cardiology to obtain such information. Instead, we will provide the reader with the tools to identify those features of the history and physical examination reported in the literature which are the most reliable and valid in assessing a patient with cardiovascular disease. We will focus on strategies to locate literature on the clinical examination, as well as guidelines to assess the quality of those studies. These techniques will then be applied to three common features of the cardiovascular history, namely chest pain, dyspnea and syncope, as well as common features of the physical examination, including assessment of the apical impulse, the third heart sound, central venous pressure, systolic murmurs, blood pressure and arterial pulse. We would also encourage the reader to access The Rational Clinical Examination series published in the *Journal of the American Medical Association* for further reviews on various aspects of the cardiovascular physical examination.[1–9] The following topics will be covered in this chapter:

- Strategies used to locate literature on clinical examination
- How to critically appraise this literature
- Application of the above in the cardiovascular history (chest pain, dyspnea, syncope)
- Application of the above in the cardiovascular physical examination (apical impulse, central venous pressure, systolic murmurs, blood pressure, arterial pulse).

Strategies used to locate literature on clinical examination

There are no validated strategies for locating precise and accurate information on obtaining a cardiovascular history and conducting a physical examination. A proposed strategy for searching the MEDLINE database is summarized in Box 2.1. This is the method suggested for authors of the Rational Clinical Examination series appearing in the *Journal of the American Medical Association.*[10] The first terms capture the clinical topic of interest by specifying the disease or presentation or function/dysfunction being sought. The second group of terms seeks clinical skills articles. The third group of terms is intended to find articles of high methodologic quality. An efficient strategy to locate high-quality articles would be to combine the first two groups of terms with "diagnosis (pre-exploded)" to maximize sensitivity, or with "sensitivity (textword)" to maximize specificity. This is an extension of the method suggested by the ACP Journal Club for finding high-quality articles on diagnostic tests in general.[11]

Box 2.1 Search strategy for clinical skills articles using MEDLINE

Group 1 terms

Term(s) for clinical entity of interest (for example, syncope, myocardial infarction) combined with (AND)*

Group 2 terms

- Physical examination (exploded; in title, abstract or subject heading)
- Medical history-taking (exploded)
- Professional competence (exploded)
- Diagnostic tests, routine
- Combined with (OR)*

Group 3 terms

- Sensitivity and specificity (textword; exploded)
- Reproducibility of results
- Observer variation
- Decision support techniques
- Bayes' theorem

*AND and OR represent Boolean terms (symbolic representation of relationships between sets) for combining items.

Any comprehensive search for relevant articles should include a review of reference lists from the articles found and review articles on the topic, as well as textbooks on clinical examination, and advice from clinicians interested in clinical examination.

How to critically appraise the literature on clinical examination studies

Having located articles on the cardiovascular clinical examination, one must carefully review each study to establish its validity, or accuracy, prior to deciding whether the results obtained will aid in establishing or ruling out a particular diagnosis. We propose a strategy for evaluating the literature on clinical examination based on a framework developed for the *Users' Guides to the Medical Literature* series.[12] In assessing the validity of the study, and interpreting the results, the following points should be considered.

- Are the results of the clinical examination study valid?
    1. Was there an independent blind comparison with a reference (gold) standard of diagnosis?
    2. Was the clinical feature evaluated in an appropriate spectrum of patients (like those in whom it would be used in clinical practice)?
    3. Was the reference standard applied regardless of the result of the clinical feature?
    4. Were the methods of performing the clinical features described in sufficient detail to permit replication?
    5. Was there a description of the experience of the individuals doing the examination?
- What were the results?
    1. Are likelihood ratios for the results presented, or data necessary for their calculation provided?
    2. Has there been consideration given to reproducibility, precision, and disagreement?

The application of the initial five guides will help the reader determine whether the results of the study are likely to be valid. If the results are deemed to be valid, the reader can then go on to interpret the results presented, of which the likelihood ratio (LR) is the most important index in determining how good a particular diagnostic test is. The likelihood ratio is the probability that the results of a test would be expected in a patient with, as opposed to one without, the target disorder.

The application of these techniques for critically appraising the cardiovascular history and physical examination will now be described.

Clinical features in the cardiovascular history

Chest pain

There are many causes of chest pain, including both cardiac and non-cardiac conditions, as outlined in Figure 2.1.

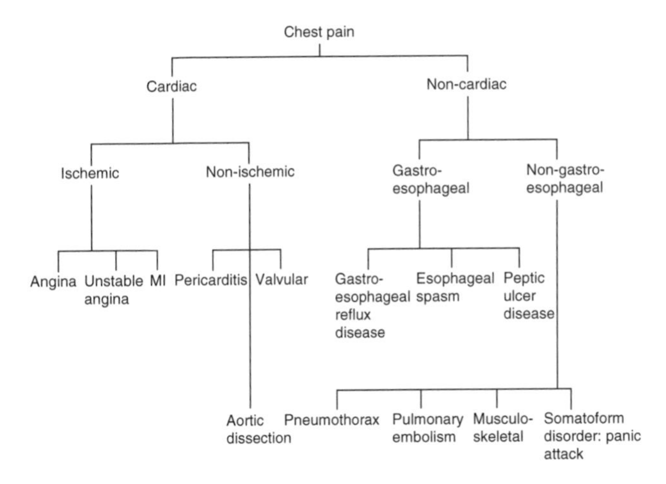

Figure 2.1 Cardiac and non-cardiac conditions presenting with chest pain

Elucidating the cause of the pain is important for both management purposes and prognosis. To ensure that the appropriate intervention is undertaken in the clinical setting, it is useful to classify patients presenting with chest pain into three categories:

1. Patients with myocardial infarction
2. Patients with myocardial ischemia but no infarction
3. Patients with non-cardiac chest pain.

The characteristics of the chest pain may help differentiate patients into the appropriate category. To identify features of the pain that might aid in classifying patients into category 1, myocardial infarction, we undertook a review of the literature using a search strategy similar to that outlined in the first section above. Relevant articles identified from this search were critically appraised using criteria outlined in the previous section. For the sake of relevance and clarity we have chosen to present only the results of those features in which a likelihood ratio of at least 2·0 or greater, or 0·5 or less, was obtained. The five studies that meet this criterion provide the best available evidence for identifying features of chest pain which aid in the diagnosis of myocardial infarction.

As outlined in Table 2.1, the features of the pain that increased the probability of a myocardial infarction included radiation, pain in the chest or left arm, and chest pain described as the most important symptom. Chest pain radiation was the clinical feature which increased the probability of a myocardial infarction the most, with a widespread distribution of pain being associated with the highest likelihood ratios. In particular, chest pain radiating to the left arm was twice as likely to occur in patients with rather than without an acute myocardial infarction, whereas radiation to the right shoulder was three times, and radiation to both the left and right arm seven times, as likely to occur in such patients. The quality of the pain, including pain described as squeezing or pressure, added little to establishing a diagnosis of myocardial infarction, with likelihood ratios of less than 2.

Table 2.1 Features of chest pain that increase the probability of a myocardial infarction

Clinical feature	References	LR (95% CI)
Chest pain radiation:		
(R) shoulder	Tierney *et al*[14]	2·9 (1·4–6·0)
(L) arm	Berger *et al*[13]	2·3 (1·7–3·1)
both (L) and (R) arm	Berger *et al*[13]	7·1 (3·6–14·2)
Pain in chest or (L) arm	Pozen *et al*[15]	2·7*
Chest pain most important symptom	Pozen *et al*[15]	2·0*

Abbreviations: CI, confidence interval; LR, likelihood ratio
*Data not available to calculate CIs.

Features of the chest pain that decrease the probability of myocardial infarction, and which therefore would be useful in ruling out a myocardial infarction, are outlined in Table 2.2. Pleuritic or positional chest pain, as well as chest pain described as sharp or stabbing, decrease the likelihood of a myocardial infarction. In addition, chest pain reproduced by palpation on physical examination was also associated with a low probability of myocardial infarction.

Table 2.2 Features of chest pain that decrease the probability of a myocardial infarction

Clinical feature	References	LR (95% CI)
Pleuritic chest pain	Tierney *et al*,[14] Lee *et al*,[16] Solomon *et al*[17]	0·2 (0·2–0·3)
Chest pain sharp or stabbing	Tierney *et al*,[14] Lee *et al*[16]	0·3 (0·2–0·5)
Positional chest pain	Lee *et al*,[16] Solomon *et al*[17]	0·3 (0·2–0·4)
Chest pain reproduced by palpation	Tierney *et al*,[14] Lee *et al*,[16] Solomon *et al*[17]	0·2–0·4*

Abbreviations: CI, confidence interval; LR, likelihood ratio
*In heterogenous studies the likelihood ratios are reported as ranges.

The precision in obtaining a chest pain history was addressed by Hickman and colleagues,[18] who assessed the interobserver agreement in chest pain histories obtained by general internists, nurse practitioners, and self-administered questionnaires for 197 inpatients and 112 outpatients with chest pain. The agreement between two internists for seven of the 10 items, including location and description of the pain, as well as aggravating and relieving factors, was substantial (κ, a measure of chance-corrected agreement, was 0·50–0·89). Agreement was slightly lower between internist and questionnaire, and between the nurse practitioners and internists, with the lowest level of agreement between nurse and questionnaire. Features of the chest pain associated with a lower probability of myocardial infarction, namely pleuritic, positional and sharp chest pain, were typically associated with a modest level of agreement for all comparisons (κ 0·26–0·62).

Although cardiac catheterization remains the definitive diagnostic procedure for allocating patients to category 2 – that is, the presence of myocardial ischemia or coronary artery disease – the character of the chest pain has also been identified as one of the most important clinical features in establishing the diagnosis of coronary artery disease.[19] The combination of typical angina and a long duration of symptoms was particularly predictive of severe disease. Although this study was undertaken in a very select group of patients (those who underwent cardiac catheterization), similar results were obtained from outpatients referred for non-invasive testing.[20] After smoking, typical angina was the variable most strongly associated with significant coronary disease (defined as >75% luminal narrowing of at least one major coronary artery). Subjects with typical angina were 13 times more likely to have significant coronary disease than those without.

There are many causes of non-cardiac chest pain, as outlined in Figure 2.1, and each condition has its own characteristic features and associated symptoms. It is beyond the scope of this chapter to identify all these conditions.

Dyspnea

Dyspnea, defined as an uncomfortable awareness of breathing, is a common complaint of both in- and outpatients. Cardiac and pulmonary causes of dyspnea are most common, with congestive heart failure, asthma and chronic obstructive pulmonary disease accounting for most complaints.[21] However, standard textbooks of internal medicine list over 30 different etiologies for dyspnea,[22] often with multiple etiologies explaining a patient's symptoms. It is often taught that the cause of dyspnea, of either the heart or the lungs, can be differentiated at the bedside by thorough history-taking. Unfortunately, such strategies to diagnose a cardiac cause for the breathless patient have been incompletely studied.

Zema and coworkers[23] looked at the value of symptoms as predictors of left ventricular systolic dysfunction in 37 patients with a clinical diagnosis of chronic obstructive pulmonary disease (COPD). Eliciting a symptom of dyspnea on exertion predicted depressed left ventricular systolic function with a sensitivity of 100% and a specificity of 20%. The symptom of orthopnea generated a sensitivity and specificity of 71% and 65%, paroxysmal nocturnal dyspnea 47% and 75%, and ankle edema 41% and 75%, respectively. All features were associated with a likelihood ratio of 2 or less. In general the study was well conducted, but the value of the results to the practicing clinician must be questioned. First, the symptoms of shortness of breath attributed to the heart were only considered in the context of impaired left ventricular (LV) systolic function. It is now generally agreed that abnormalities in LV diastolic function also cause symptoms of dyspnea. A better gold standard would perhaps have been radionuclide ventriculographic evidence of both LV systolic and diastolic dysfunction. The generalizability of the results is also lessened by the fact that their definition of heart failure was a left ventricular ejection fraction (LVEF) <50%, when in fact the target for treatment of patients with heart failure is most often an LVEF of <40%. Finally, the study was performed in patients who first had a clinical diagnosis of COPD, when patients present with many causes of shortness of breath, not just COPD.

In summary, therefore, specific features when elicited in a patient presenting with a complaint of dyspnea are of limited usefulness in making a definitive diagnosis of impaired LV function.

Syncope

Little detailed evidence exists for either individual or clusters of clinical examination findings in the evaluation of syncope. In a prospective study of 433 syncopal patients presenting in a university setting (emergency, in- and outpatients), the history and physical examination were found to identify 55% (140) of the 254 causes ultimately found.[24] Many of the non-cardiac causes of syncope in this study were defined in clinical terms, and so provided the "diagnostic standard" for classification. The three most common non-cardiac causes were "orthostatic hypotension" (systolic drop of more than 25 mmHg, or drop of more than 10 mmHg to less than 90 mmHg with symptoms), "situational" (situations included cough, micturition and defecation, and required appropriate timing and no other identifiable cause) and "vasovagal" (requiring a precipitating event and premonitory symptoms), representing 31%, 26% and 25%, respectively, of identifiable causes of syncope overall.

Follow-up of the cohort demonstrated a 5 year mortality of 50·5% for cardiac versus 30% for non-cardiac or 24% for unknown causes. This provides some independent validation for the clinical classification criteria.

There is a need for further work in this area, particularly in developing and validating practical clinical tools to screen for psychiatric causes, to distinguish patients who will benefit from electrophysiologic testing, and to predict those who will have a positive tilt-table test.

Clinical features in the cardiovascular physical examination

Apical impulse

The apical impulse was first described by William Harvey in 1928[25] and is one of a number of palpable precordial pulsations reflecting the underlying movement of the heart and great vessels. Many criteria exist defining the normal location, size and character of the apical impulse, and many generations of medical students have been taught that an "abnormal" apical impulse may assist with the diagnosis of left ventricular enlargement and/or hypertrophy. It is only recently that evidence has been published to support these claims.

The relationship between the location and size of the apical impulse and LV size, as determined by two-dimensional echocardiography (gold standard), was evaluated by Eilen and colleagues.[26] An apical impulse lateral to the midclavicular line, defined as half the distance between the tip of the acromion process and the sternal notch, was a sensitive (100%) but not specific (18%) indicator for LV enlargement, with a likelihood ratio of only 1·2. Identification of the apical impulse <10 cm from the midsternal line was just as sensitive (100%) but only marginally more specific (33%). An apical diameter of <3 cm was a good indicator of LV enlargement, with a sensitivity of 92% and a specificity of 75%, and was almost four times as likely to occur in patients with, as opposed to those without, LV enlargement (LR=3·7).

O'Neill and coworkers[27] examined the relationship between the location of the apical impulse and the presence or absence of cardiomegaly on chest *x*-ray (defined as a cardiothoracic ratio greater than 50%). An apical impulse lateral to the midclavicular line had a sensitivity of 57%, a specificity of 76%, and a likelihood ratio of 2·4 for identifying cardiomegaly. Identification of the apical impulse >10 cm from the midsternal line was slightly more sensitive (78%) but considerably less specific (28%), and added little to establishing the diagnosis (LR=1·1). The results of this investigation must be accepted with caution, as the gold standard used in this case was chest *x*-ray, which is not a sensitive or specific marker of LV enlargement. Therefore, the validity of this gold standard must be questioned. This was, however, one of the few studies that also evaluated the variation between observers (interobserver variation) in the clinical assessment of the apical impulse, and reported good agreement on apex palpability (κ=0·72) and moderate agreement on degree of apex displacement (κ=0·56) between two physicians.

Eagle and coworkers[28] examined several clinical features in 125 inpatients with a variety of cardiac and non-cardiac diagnoses in an attempt to determine which features best predicted LVEF. In general, physician estimates of LVEF were good, with 56% being accurate within 7·5% of measured value; 27% of physicians overestimated and 17% underestimated the LVEF. Multiple regression analysis identified three clinical features most predictive of LVEF, including S_3 gallop, hypotension, and sustained LV apical impulse (defined as a palpable impulse greater than two thirds the ventricle systole).

In summary, the location, size and character of the apical impulse may be used to assess LV size, LV function and cardiomegaly, either alone or in combination with other clinical features or simple diagnostic tests. However, a number of limitations exist, including the fact that a palpable impulse may only be found in approximately 50% of patients. In addition, the high sensitivity but low specificity associated with determining the location and size of the apical impulse make it a better test for ruling out rather than ruling in LV enlargement, which is good for screening but has limited usefulness at the bedside.

Third heart sound

Few studies have assessed the reliability and validity of detecting a third heart sound on physical examination. The studies that have been conducted suggest that the agreement between observers with respect to the presence of a third heart sound is low or moderate at best.[29–31] In one study, cardiologists, internists and residents in internal medicine examined 46 patients for the presence or absence of a third heart sound.[30] The overall interobserver agreement was poor, with a κ of only 0·18. A somewhat better agreement for the presence of a third heart sound was achieved in an earlier study by two internists and two cardiologists, with a κ of 0·40.[31] The evidence regarding the validity of the third heart sound is even more limited. Using a computerized phonocardiogram as a gold standard for the presence of a third heart sound, Lok *et al*[30] report positive and negative predictive values for identifying a third heart sound of 71% and 64%, respectively.

Although the reliability and validity of this physical examination finding may be limited, the detection of a third heart sound on physical examination may have important prognostic implications. Drazner and colleagues[32] performed a retrospective analysis of 2569 patients with symptomatic heart failure enrolled in the Studies of Left Ventricular Dysfunction treatment trial. In multivariate analyses adjusted for other markers of severity of heart failure, a third heart sound was associated with an almost 50% increased risk of hospitalization for heart failure, or death from pump failure.

Central venous pressure

The right internal jugular vein lies directly in line with the right atrium and acts as a manometer, displaying changes in blood flow and pressure caused by right atrial filling, contraction and emptying. Elevated jugular venous pressure reflects an increase in central venous pressure (CVP).

The reliability and validity of the clinical assessment of CVP have been assessed in a limited number of studies. In one study, medical students, residents and attending physicians examined the same 50 ICU patients and estimated their CVP as low (<5 cm), normal (5–10 cm) or high (>10 cm).[33] Agreement between students and residents was substantial (κ 0·65), agreement between students and attending physicians was moderate (κ 0·56), and agreement between residents and staff was modest (κ 0·30). Possible causes for disagreement include positioning of patients, poor lighting, difficulty in distinguishing carotid from venous pulsations, and variation in pressure with respiration.

As regards the relation between clinical assessments of CVP and the gold standard of simultaneous pressure measurements through a central venous catheter, one study[34] used an attending physician, a fellow, a medical resident, an intern and a student to predict whether four hemodynamic variables, including CVP, were low, normal, high or very high. The sensitivity of the clinical examination at identifying low (<0 mmHg), normal (0–7 mmHg) or high (>7 mmHg) CVP was 33%, 33% and 49%, respectively. The specificity of the clinical examination at identifying low, normal or high CVP was 73%, 62% and 76%, respectively. In another study, Eisenberg and colleagues[35] compared clinical assessments with pulmonary artery catheter readings in 97 critically ill patients. Physicians predicted CVP correctly only 55% of the time, more frequently (27%) underestimating than overestimating (17%).

Clinical assessments of a high CVP increase the likelihood that the measured CVP will be high by about fourfold; conversely, clinical assessments of a low CVP make the probability of finding a high measured CVP extremely unlikely (LR= 0·2).[33] The data demonstrate that clinical assessments of a normal CVP are truly indeterminate, with likelihood ratios approaching 1; such estimates provide no information because they neither increase nor decrease the probability of an abnormal CVP. Apart from less observer variation, CVP estimates are most accurate in patients breathing spontaneously.

The precision of the abdominojugular reflux test has not been reported, but its results will vary with the force of abdominal compression. Although this is an insensitive way to diagnose congestive heart failure, the specificity of the test is high.[36,37] Moreover, the positive likelihood ratios (6·4 when diagnosis was based on a clinical–radiographic score, and 6·0 when diagnosis was based on emergency room physician judgment) indicate that this is a useful bedside test.[1]

Systolic murmurs

Etchells and colleagues[2] have published a thorough review of the clinical examination for systolic murmurs. This included a systematic review of the literature and grading of the quality of the original articles. Quality was assessed by the sample size and recruitment (consecutive versus convenience) and whether comparison with the diagnostic standard was done independently and blindly.

Useful data for ruling aortic stenosis in or out are given in Tables 2.3 and 2.4. The reliability of the examination by cardiologists for late peaking murmur shape is good (κ 0·74), for the presence of murmurs is fair to moderate (κ 0·29–0·48),[2] but for other maneuvers may be poorer.[38]

Table 2.3 Features of the clinical examination that increase the probability of aortic stenosis

Clinical feature	LR*
Slow rate of rise of carotid pulse	2·8–130
Late peaking murmur	8–101
Soft or absent second heart sound	3·1–50

*LR, likelihood ratio: range of point estimates from original studies cited
Data from Etchells *et al*[2]

Table 2.4 Features of the clinical examination that decrease the probability of aortic stenosis

Clinical feature	LR*
Absence of a murmur	0
No radiation to right carotid artery	0·05–0·10

*LR, likelihood ratio: range of point estimates from original studies cited
Data from Etchells *et al*[2]

Studies of the clinical examination for other etiologies of systolic murmur were also reviewed but tended to be of lesser quality than those addressing aortic stenosis.

Subsequent to their original work,[2] Etchells and colleagues have gone on to develop a two-stage prediction rule for moderate–severe aortic stenosis (defined as an average valve area of less than or equal to 1·2 cm^2 or a peak gradient at or above 25 mmHg).[39] In this rule a murmur not radiating to the right clavicle was associated with a likelihood ratio of 0·1 (95% CI 0·02–0·44), significantly reducing the likelihood of aortic stenosis. If the murmur did radiate to the clavicle, the presence of 0–2 associated findings increased the likelihood ratio to 1·76 (95% CI 0·9–2·9), and 3–4 associated findings resulted in a likelihood ratio of 40 (95% CI 6·6–239), suggesting that the diagnosis of aortic stenosis is supported by a greater number of associated findings. The associated findings were reduced carotid volume, slow carotid upstroke, reduced second heart sound intensity, and murmur intensity in the second right intercostal space as loud as or louder than in the fifth left intercostal space.

Etchells and colleagues[2] point out that the majority of studies of this topic have used cardiologists as observers. The performance of non-cardiologists appears to be less accurate when studied. Further work, like their own, using a broader range of clinicians and patients, is needed to discover the value of the clinical examination in more general settings.

Blood pressure

An extensive review of the technique, reliability and validity of blood pressure (BP) measurement has been provided by Reeves.[3] As outlined in the review, two important sources of variation in BP measurement include the patient and the examiner. Random fluctuation in BP over time has been documented by the SD of readings, with a minute-to-minute variation of about 4 mmHg systolic and 2–3 mmHg diastolic, and day to day variation of 5–12 mmHg systolic and 6–8 mmHg diastolic. With respect to the examiner as the source of variability, differences of 10–8 mmHg by both physicians and nurses in routine medical practices have been noted.

Intra-arterial blood pressure measurement has been used as the gold standard to assess the accuracy of indirect BP measurement. With the indirect BP the phase I Korotkoff, or first audible sound, appears 15–4 mmHg below the direct systolic BP, whereas phase V, or disappearance of all sounds, appears 3–6 mmHg above the true diastolic BP in adults. Other factors that affect the accuracy of the indirect BP measurement, resulting in both an increase and a decrease in systolic and/or diastolic measurements, are outlined in Tables 2.5 and 2.6.

Table 2.5 Factors associated with an increase in blood pressure

Factor	Magnitude, SBP/DBP (mmHg)
Examinee	
Pseudohypertension	2–98/3–49
"White coat reaction" to physician	11–28/3–15
"White coat reaction" to non-physician	1–12/2–7
Paretic arm (due to stroke)	2/5
Pain, anxiety	May be large
Acute smoking	6/5
Acute caffeine	11/5
Acute ethanol ingestion	8/8
Distended bladder	15/10
Talking, sighing	7/8
Setting, equipment	
Leaky bulb valve	>2 DBP
Blocked manometer vents	2 to 10
Examination	
Cuff too narrow	−8–+10/2–8
Cuff not centered	4/3
Cuff over clothing	5–50
Elbow too low	6
Back unsupported	6–10
Arm unsupported	1–7/5–11
Too slow deflation	−1–+2/5–6
Too fast deflation	DBP only
Parallax error	2–4
Using phase IV (adult)	6 DBP
Too rapid remeasure	1/1
Cold season (*v* warm)	6/3–10

Abbreviations: DBP, diastolic blood pressure; SBP, systolic blood pressure
Data from Reeves *et al*[3]

Table 2.6 Factors associated with a decrease in blood pressure

Factor	Magnitude, SBP/DBP (mmHg)
Examinee	
Recent meal	−1−1/1−4
Missed auscultatory gap	10–50 SBP
High stroke volume	Phase V can=0
Habituation	0–7/2–12
Shock (additional pseudohypotension)	33 SBP
Setting, equipment	
Faulty aneroid device	Can be >10
Leaky bulb	≥2 SBP
Examiner	
Reading to next lowest 5 or 10 mmHg or expectation bias	Probably ≤10
Impaired hearing	SBP only
Examination	
Left *v* right arm	1/1
Resting for too long (25 min)	10/0
Elbow too high	5/5
Too rapid deflation	SBP only
Excess bell pressure	≥9 DBP
Parallax error (aneroid)	2–4

Abbreviations: DBP, diastolic blood pressure; SBP, systolic blood pressure
Data from Reeves *et al*[3]

Arterial pulse

Few studies have been undertaken to assess the reliability and validity of features of the arterial pulse in the cardiovascular examination, despite numerous descriptive accounts of its variability in different clinical conditions. Case series indicate that details regarding the presence and quality of the arterial pulse are more sensitive markers of coarctation of the aorta than aortic dissection. Absent femoral pulses or a femoral/brachial pulse discrepancy in patients was associated with a sensitivity of 88% in the diagnosis of coarctation of the aorta in patients less than 6 months of age.[40] Similar results were obtained for patients diagnosed with coarctation after 1 year of age, where weak or absent femoral pulses were associated with a sensitivity of 85%.[41]

The sensitivity of the presence and quality of the carotid, subclavian and femoral pulses in establishing a diagnosis of both proximal (primary tear in the ascending aorta with or without involvement of the arch, De Bakey classification type I and II) and distal (primary tear in the descending thoracic aorta, De Bakey classification type III) aortic dissections are outlined in Table 2.7. Proximal dissections were primarily associated with an absence or decrease in the brachiocephalic vessels, whereas distal dissections almost exclusively involved the femoral arteries.

Table 2.7 Sensitivity of the arterial pulse in the diagnosis of aortic dissection

	Aortic dissection (%)	
References	Proximal*	Distal†
Lindsay and Hurst[42§]	62·5	10·5
Slater and De Sanctis[43§]	50·9	15·5
Spittell *et al*[44**]	9·0	2·4

*De Bakey classification type I and II.
†De Bakey classification type III.
§Absence or decrease in amplitude of carotid, subclavian or femoral pulse(s).
**Absence of palpable carotid, subclavian or femoral pulse(s).

Features of the arterial pulse may also be used to determine the presence of valvular heart disease. As reported by Etchells *et al*,[2] features of the arterial pulse, including rate of rise of the carotid pulse, apical carotid delay and brachioradial delay, all increase the likelihood of establishing the diagnosis of aortic stenosis (Table 2.8).

Table 2.8 Features of the arterial pulse that increase the probability of aortic stenosis

Clinical feature	LR*
Slow rate of rise of carotid pulse	2·8–130
Apical carotid delay	∞
Brachioradial delay	6·8

*LR, likelihood ratio: range of point estimates from original studies cited.
Data from Etchells *et al*[2]

The diagnostic value of the pedal pulse examination, as an aid to establishing the diagnosis of peripheral arterial disease, has also been studied.[45] In this review the absence of both the dorsalis pedis and posterior tibial pulses was a powerful predictor for the presence of vascular disease (defined as an ankle-to-arm systolic pressure index of <0·9), with likelihood ratios ranging from 9·0 to 44·6. The presence of a femoral arterial bruit was also a strong indicator of disease, with likelihood ratios of 4·7–5·7.

Heart rate is another important component of the cardiovascular examination. The accuracy of the assessment of heart rate may be affected by both the site (apical or radial) as well as the counting interval (15, 30 or 60 seconds). With a regular rhythm, radial 15 second counts were the least accurate for both resting and rapid heart rates, whereas the 30 second counts were found to be the most accurate and efficient for rapid rates.[46] With the irregularly irregular rhythm of atrial fibrillation, however, the apical method and 60 second count have been reported to be the most accurate, with site being a more important source of error than counting interval.[47] Using the ECG as the measure of true heart rate, the mean radial error for all counting intervals was 19·5 beats per minute, which was significantly higher than the mean apical error of 9·7 beats per minute.

Although the pulse in atrial fibrillation is typically described as "irregularly irregular", Rawles and Rowland,[48] using computerized analysis of R–R intervals and pulse volumes in patients with atrial fibrillation, disputed this assumption. In an assessment of 74 patients with atrial fibrillation they reported a non-random sequence of R–R intervals in 30%, and the presence of pulsus alternans in less than half (46%). The authors concluded that patterns of regularity of the pulse are common in patients with atrial fibrillation.

Summary

Despite the frequency with which details of the history and physical examination are used to establish or rule out a particular cardiovascular condition, there is a very limited amount of data available to support the reliability and validity of these features. The one component of the cardiovascular history which has been studied is that of chest pain in the diagnosis of myocardial infarction. Features of chest pain, particularly pain that has a wide distribution of radiation, increase the probability of myocardial infarction, whereas chest pain that is pleuritic, sharp or stabbing, positional or reproduced by palpation, decreases the probability of myocardial infarction.

The reliability and validity of various features of the cardiovascular physical examination have also received little attention in the literature. Of those that have been studied, the apical impulse has been shown to be a sensitive but nonspecific marker of LV size, which makes it useful for ruling out, rather than ruling in, LV enlargement. Clinical assessment of elevated CVP has been shown to be associated with a fourfold likelihood that the measured CVP will be high, with the abdominojugular reflex being a useful bedside test to assist in the diagnosis of congestive heart failure.

Of the cardiac murmurs, aortic stenosis has been studied the most thoroughly. Features of the clinical examination that increase the probability of diagnosing aortic stenosis include slow rate of rise of the carotid pulse, late peaking murmur, and soft or absent second heart sound. Conversely, absence of a murmur or no radiation to the right carotid artery or clavicle were features associated with a decreased probability of aortic stenosis. Recent work would suggest that the presence of an increased number of associated findings increases the likelihood of aortic stenosis.

A number of features have been shown to influence the accuracy of the indirect assessment of BP, including those related to the examinee, the examiner, the setting and equipment, and the examination itself. Assessment of the arterial pulse in diagnosing coarctation of the aorta and aortic dissection has been limited to case series, therefore estimates of sensitivity only are available. Features of the arterial pulse have been shown to be relatively sensitive markers for coarctation of the aorta and for chronic lower extremity ischemia, but less so for aortic dissection. Finally, both counting interval and site (radial versus apical) have important implications on the accuracy of heart rate assessment.

As is evident from the information presented, unfortunately, for a variety of reasons, research on clinical examination has lagged behind basic science and therapeutic research. So far, clinical examination is identified as the "art" of medicine, and by incorporating an evidence-based approach one can make clinical examination the "art and science" of medicine.

References

1. Cook DJ, Simel DL. Does this patient have abnormal central venous pressure? *JAMA* 1996;**275**:630–4.
2. Etchells E, Bell C, Robb K. Does this patient have an abnormal systolic murmur? *JAMA* 1997;**277**:564–71.
3. Reeves RA. Does this patient have hypertension? *JAMA* 1995; **273**:1211–18.
4. Choudhry NK, Etchells EE. Does this patient have aortic regurgitation? *JAMA* 1999;**281**:2231–8.
5. Panju AA, Hemmelgarn BR, Guyatt GH, Simel DL. Is this patient having a myocardial infarction? *JAMA* 1998;**280**: 1256–63.
6. Turnbull JM. Is listening for abdominal bruits useful in the evaluation of hypertension? *JAMA* 1995;**274**:1299–301.
7. Badgett RG, Lucey CR, Mulrow CD *et al.* Can the clinical examination diagnose left-sided heart failure? *JAMA* 1997; **277**:1712–19.
8. Lederle FA, Simel DL. Does this patient have abdominal aortic aneurysm? *JAMA* 1999;**281**:77–82.
9. McGee S, Abernathy WB, Simel DL. Is this patient hypovolemic? *JAMA* 1999;**281**:1022–9.
10. Simel D (Section editor, Rational Clinical Examination, *JAMA*). Personal communication, December 1996.
11. McKibbon KA, Walker-Dilks CJ. Beyond ACP Journal Club: How to harness MEDLINE for diagnostic problems (Editorial). *ACP J Club* 1994;**121**:A10–A12.
12. Oxman AD, Sackett DL, Guyatt GH. Users' Guides to the Medical Literature: 1. How to get started. *JAMA* 1993;**270**: 2093–5.
13. Berger JP, Buclin R, Haller E, Van Melle G, Yersin B. Right arm involvement and pain extension can help to differentiate coronary diseases from chest pain of other origin: a prospective emergency ward study of 278 consecutive patients admitted for chest pain. *J Intern Med* 1990;**227**:165–72.
14. Tierney WM, Fitzgerald D, McHenry R *et al.* Physicians' estimates of the probability of myocardial infarction in emergency room patients with chest pain. *Med Decis Making* 1986;**6**:12–17.
15. Pozen MW, D'Agostino RB, Selker HP, Sytkowski PA, Hood WB. A predictive instrument to improve coronary-care-unit

admission practices in acute ischemic heart disease. *N Engl J Med* 1984;**310**:1273–8.
16.Lee TH, Cook EF, Weisberg M *et al.* Acute chest pain in the emergency room. *Arch Intern Med* 1985;**145**:65–9.
17.Solomon CG, Lee TH, Cook EF *et al.* Comparison of clinical presentation of acute myocardial infarction in patients older than 65 years of age to younger patients: the multicenter chest pain study experience. *Am J Cardiol* 1989;**63**:772–6.
18.Hickman DH, Sox HC, Sox CH. Systematic bias in recording the history in patients with chest pain. *J Chron Dis* 1985; **38**:91–100.
19.Pryor DB, Shaw L, Harrell FE *et al.* Estimating the likelihood of severe coronary artery disease. *Am J Med* 1991;**90**:553–62.
20.Pryor DB, Shaw L, McCants CB. Value of the history and physical in identifying patients at increased risk for coronary artery disease. *Ann Intern Med* 1993;**118**:81–90.
21.Mulrow CD, Lucey CR, Farnett LE. Discriminating causes of dyspnea through clinical examination. *J Gen Intern Med* 1993;**8**:383–92.
22.Ingram RH Jr, Braunwald E. Dyspnea and pulmonary edema. In: Wilson JD *et al.*, eds. Harrison's principles of internal medicine, 12th edn. New York: McGraw-Hill, 1991.
23.Zema MJ, Masters AP, Malgouleff D. Dyspnea: the heart or the lungs? Differentiation at bedside by use of the simple valsalva maneuver. *Chest* 1984;**85**:59–64.
24.Kapoor WN. Evaluation and outcome of patients with syncope. *Medicine* 1990;**69**:160–75.
25.Harvey W. *An anatomical disquisition on the motion of the heart and blood in animals.* London, 1928. (Translated from the Latin by Robert Willis, Barnes, Surrey, England, 1847.) In: Willius FA, Key TE. *Classics of cardiology*, vol. 1. Malabar, Florida: Robert E. Krieger, 1983.
26.Eilen SD, Crawford MH, O'Rourke RA. Accuracy of precordial palpation for detecting increased left ventricular volume. *Ann Intern Med* 1983;**99**:628–30.
27.O'Neill TW, Barry M, Smith M, Graham IM. Diagnostic value of the apex beat. *Lancet* 1989;**i**:410–11.
28.Eagle KA, Quertermous T, Singer DE *et al.* Left ventricular ejection fraction. Physician estimates compared with gated blood pool scan measurements. *Arch Intern Med* 1988;**148**:882–5
29.Westman EC, Matchar DB, Samsa GP, Mulrow CD, Waugh RA, Feussner JR. Accuracy and reliability of apical S3 gallop detection. *J Gen Intern Med* 1995;**10**:455–7.
30.Lok CE, Morgan CD, Ranganathan N. The accuracy and interobserver agreement in detecting the "gallop sounds" by cardiac auscultation. *Chest* 1998;**114**:1283–8.
31.Ishmail AA, Wing S, Ferguson J, Hutchinson TA, Magder S, Flegel KM. Interobserver agreement by auscultation in the presence of a third heart sound in patients with congestive heart failure. *Chest* 1987;**91**:870–3.
32.Drazner MH, Rame JE, Phil M, Stevenson LW, Dries DL. Prognostic importance of elevated jugular venous pressure and a third heart sound in patients with heart failure. *N Engl J Med* 2001;**345**:574–81.
33.Cook DJ. The clinical assessment of central venous pressure. *Am J Med Sci* 1990;**299**:175–8.
34.Connors AF, McCaffree DR, Gray BA. Evaluation of right heart catheterization in the critically ill patient without acute myocardial infarction. *N Engl J Med* 1983;**308**:263–7.
35.Eisenberg PR, Jaffe AS, Schuster DP. Clinical evaluation compared to pulmonary artery catheterization in the hemodynamic assessment of critically ill patients. *Crit Care Med* 1984;**12**:549–53.
36.Marantz PR, Kaplan MC, Alderman MH. Clinical diagnosis of congestive heart failure in patients with acute dyspnea. *Chest* 1990;**97**:776–81.
37.Maisel AS, Atwood JE, Goldberger AL. Hepatojugular reflux: useful in the bedside diagnosis of tricuspid regurgitation. *Ann Intern Med* 1984;**101**:781–2.
38.Spodick DH, Sugiura T, Doi Y, Paladion D, Jaffty BG. Rate of rise of the carotid pulse: an investigation of observer error in a common clinical measurement. *Am J Cardiol* 1982;**49**:159–62.
39.Etchells E, Glenns V, Shadowitz S, Bell C, Siu S. A bedside clinical prediction rule for detecting moderate or severe aortic stenosis. *J Gen Intern Med* 1998;**13**:699–704.
40.Ward KE, Pryor RW, Matson JR *et al.* Delayed detection of coarctation in infancy: implications for timing of newborn follow-up. *Pediatrics* 1990;**86**:972–6.
41.Strafford MA, Griffiths SP, Gersony WM. Coarctation of the aorta: a study in delayed detection. *Pediatrics* 1982;**69**:159–63.
42.Lindsay J, Hurst JW. Clinical features and prognosis in dissecting aneurysm of the aorta. *Circulation* 1967;**35**:880–8.
43.Slater EE, DeSanctis RW. The clinical recognition of dissecting aortic aneurysm. *Am J Med* 1976;**60**:625–33.
44.Spittell PC, Spittell JA, Joyce JW *et al.* Clinical features and differential diagnosis of aortic dissection: experience with 236 cases (1980 through 1990). *Mayo Clin Proc* 1993;**68**:642–51.
45.McGee SR, Boyko EJ. Physical examination and chronic lower-extremity ischemia. *Arch Intern Med* 1998;**158**:1357–64.
46.Hollerbach AD, Sneed NV. Accuracy of radial pulse assessment by length of counting interval. *Heart Lung* 1990;**19**: 258–64.
47.Sneed NV, Hollerbach AD. Accuracy of heart rate assessment in atrial fibrillation. *Heart Lung* 1992;**21**:427–33.
48.Rawles JM, Rowland E. Is the pulse in atrial fibrillation irregularly irregular? *Br Heart J* 1986;**56**:4–11.

3 Obtaining incremental information from diagnostic tests

Raymond J Gibbons

Consider the following case history. A 75 year old male presents with a history of exertional chest pain. The patient describes substernal chest pain that he perceives as a "pressure sensation" occurring when he walks too fast, uphill, or in the cold. It is relieved by rest within a few minutes. On two recent occasions, he tried a friend's nitroglycerin tablets, and obtained even more rapid relief of his symptoms. His symptoms have never occurred at rest. The patient has a history of diabetes mellitus, hypertension, and hypercholesterolemia. He smokes one pack of cigarettes a day. Several male family members died of coronary artery disease before the age of 60. The patient underwent carotid artery surgery a year ago for treatment of transient ischemic attacks.

On the basis of his age, gender, chest pain description, and risk factors, this patient is highly likely to have significant obstructive coronary artery disease (CAD). The added, or incremental, value of any stress test for the diagnosis of the presence of disease in such a situation is very small. Out of 100 patients with this presentation, perhaps only one or two will not have obstructive CAD. The potential contribution of stress testing is therefore restricted to only these one or two patients.

This example demonstrates the importance of the concept of incremental value for diagnostic tests. In the current era of healthcare reform, it is no longer sufficient that a test simply provide "more information". The more appropriate current questions are:

- how much information does the test provide, and
- at what cost?

Increasingly, tests are also required to have a demonstrable impact on critical nodal, or decision, points with respect to patient management.

The demonstration of the incremental value of diagnostic tests requires rigorous methodology. The principles of the required methodology should be credited primarily to Dr George Diamond and his colleagues at Cedar Sinai Medical Center in Los Angeles.[1–3] First and foremost, such an analysis should reflect clinical decision making. Since clinical assessment is performed before any diagnostic tests, and usually at lower cost, parameters available from this assessment should be considered separately without any information from subsequent testing. The analysis should preferably focus on hard, demonstrable end points such as significant obstructive CAD, severe (three vessel or left main) coronary artery disease, myocardial infarction, or death. Although alternative end points, such as functional impairment, unstable angina, and the need for revascularization, are often included to increase statistical power, such end points have major limitations with respect to reversibility, subjectivity, and definite impact on patient outcome. The analysis should create appropriate models that include all available important variables. An experienced clinician always takes the patient's age, gender, and history into account in making his or her clinical decision regarding patient management, even when testing results are available. These important clinical parameters must therefore be included in any final model that reflects the clinical decision making process. The analysis must demonstrate that the additional information is statistically significant in an appropriate patient population. Analyses that demonstrate additional information in older, "sicker" inpatient populations should not be casually extrapolated to younger, "less sick" outpatients in whom testing is customarily performed. Finally, the test must provide information that is clinically significant and cost effective. In very large patient samples, differences that have little, if any, clinical significance for individual patient management may emerge as statistically significant. The potential impact on patient management in *some* patients must compare favorably with the incremental cost of the test in *all* the patients who must be tested.

This chapter will attempt to elucidate this methodology using the published data with respect to the diagnosis of significant obstructive CAD, non-invasive screening for severe CAD, and patient outcome. All of these examples are drawn from the arena of ischemic heart disease, because this entity is a predominant feature of clinical practice in cardiology, and the published literature is voluminous and extensive. However, the same principles apply to other disease entities, both cardiac and non-cardiac.

Clinical assessment

As outlined above, the initial step in any analysis designed to demonstrate incremental value is the consideration of all the information available prior to performance of the test. This will always include the results of the history and physical examination, and may sometimes include the results of other tests already performed. This section focuses on the information available from clinical assessment.

Diagnosis of coronary disease

As demonstrated by the earlier example, clinicians often encounter patients with chest pain and suspected CAD. The ability of clinical assessment to predict the likelihood of significant obstructive CAD has been demonstrated in numerous studies. The likelihood of significant disease based on clinical assessment is appropriately labeled the "pretest probability", in statistical terms.

Age, gender, and the patient's chest pain description are the most important clinical parameters for estimating the likelihood of CAD.[4] Older patients, men, and patients with chest pain that is typical, or classic, for angina pectoris are more likely to have coronary disease. Although multiple different systems have been used to classify chest pain, the simplest and easiest was proposed by Diamond.[5] He suggested a classification based on three elements – substernal location, precipitation by exertion, and relief by rest or nitroglycerin. If all three elements are present, the chest pain is classified as "typical angina". If two elements are present, the chest pain is classified as "atypical angina". If only one or none is present, the chest pain is classified as "non-anginal chest pain".

Table 3.1 shows published estimates of pretest probability on the basis of age, gender, and chest pain description.[4] It is obvious that there is a very wide range of pretest probability, ranging from 1% for a 35 year old woman with non-anginal chest pain to 94% for a 65 year old man with typical angina. Note that a 50 year old man with atypical angina has about a 50% probability of disease.

A more comprehensive attempt to consider all clinical characteristics, including risk factors for atherosclerosis, was published from the Duke University Medical Center databank.[6] In addition to the three parameters previously discussed, this analysis found that evidence for previous infarction, smoking, hyperlipidemia, ST and T wave changes on the resting electrocardiogram (ECG), and diabetes were all highly significant predictors of the presence of coronary artery disease. Figure 3.1 shows a published nomogram for men that incorporates all of these parameters. Careful inspection of this figure demonstrates that the impact of the clinical parameters other than age, gender, and chest pain is variable. ECG and historical evidence of previous infarction have a major impact, diabetes and ECG ST-T changes have a modest impact, and lipids and smoking have a minimal impact. For example, a 50 year old male with atypical angina has a 46% pretest probability of disease in the absence of smoking, hyperlipidemia, or diabetes, a 48% pretest probability in the presence of both smoking and hyperlipidemia, and a 65% pretest probability if he has diabetes as well. In the presence of ECG Q waves and a history of MI, his pretest probability exceeds 90%.

Non-invasive screening for severe coronary artery disease

Not surprisingly, clinical parameters are also very important in estimating the likelihood of severe (three vessel or left main) CAD.[7] The same parameters that are most important for predicting the presence of disease – age, gender, and chest pain description – remain important. In addition, diabetes mellitus and history or ECG evidence of myocardial infarction are also very important. The simplest approach for estimating the likelihood of severe disease was published by Hubbard *et al.*[8] They assigned one point each for: male gender; typical angina; history and ECG evidence of myocardial infarction;

Table 3.1 Pretest probability of coronary artery disease

Age (years)	Pretest probability (%)							
	Asymptomatic		Non-anginal chest pain		Atypical angina		Typical angina	
	F	M	F	M	F	M	F	M
30–39	<1	2	1	5	4	22	26	70
40–49	1	6	3	14	13	46	55	87
50–59	4	9	8	22	32	59	79	92
60–69	8	11	19	28	54	67	91	94

From Diamond and Forrester.[4] Reprinted by permission of the *New England Journal of Medicine*, and Diamond GA. A clinically relevant classification of chest discomfort. *J Am Coll Cardiol* 1983;**1**:547–75

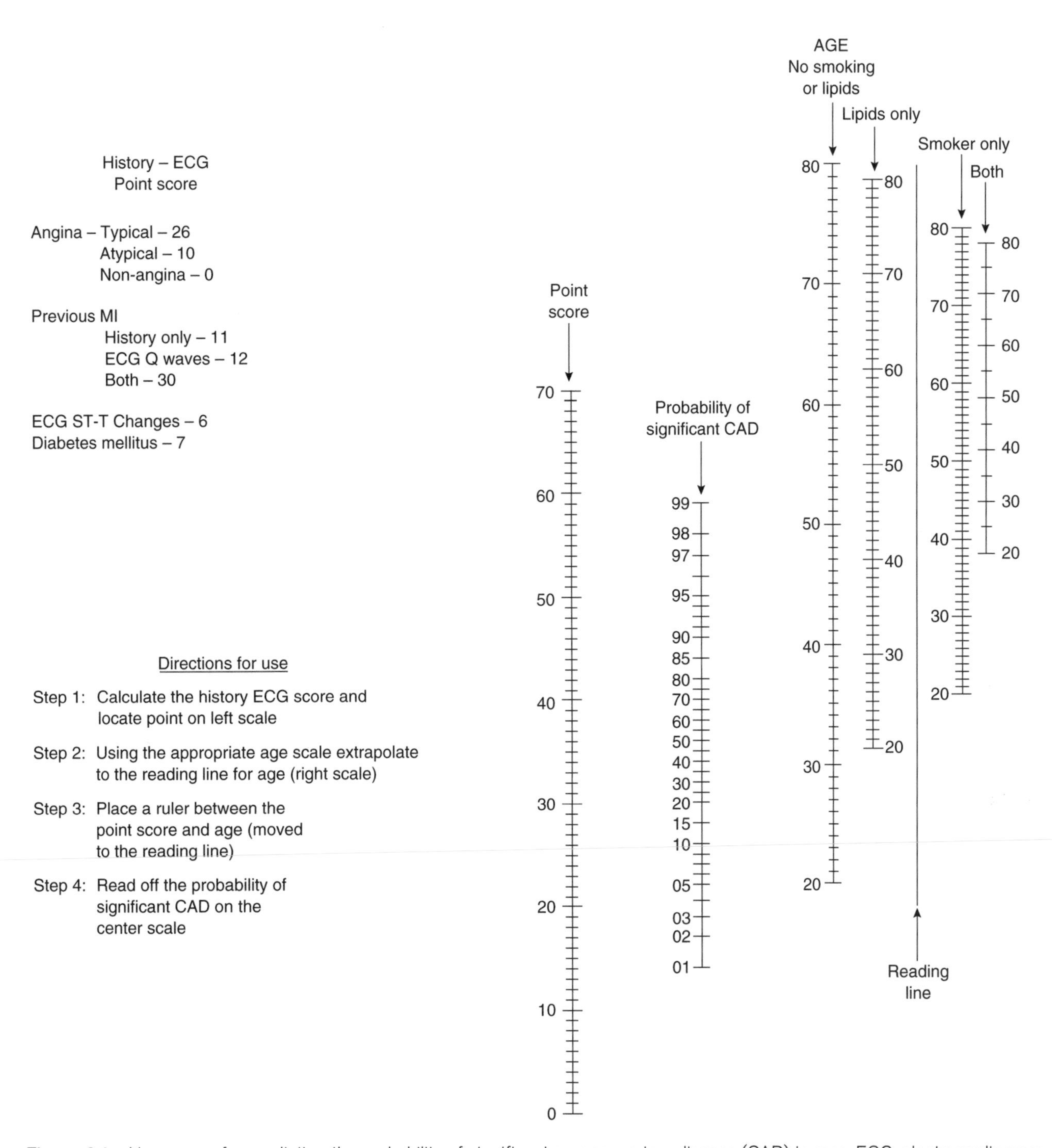

Figure 3.1 Nomogram for predicting the probability of significant coronary artery disease (CAD) in men. ECG, electrocardiogram; MI, myocardial infarction. (After Pryor *et al.*[6]) Example: A 50 year old, white male with atypical angina and diabetes mellitus, but no ECG ST changes, previous MI, smoking, or hyperlipidemia. Point score on left scale = 10 + 7 = 17. Appropriate reading line on right labeled "no smoking or lipids". Connect age 50 on this reading line to point score of 17 with a straight edge. This intersects the middle line at 60, indicating that this is the percentage probability of significant CAD.

diabetes; and insulin use. Thus, the point score had a minimum value of 0 and a maximum value of 5. Figure 3.2 shows a nomogram for the probability of severe CAD based on age and this point score. It is quickly apparent that age is an extremely important parameter for predicting severe disease.

A more comprehensive analysis on a larger number of patients was published from the Duke University Medical Center databank.[9] In addition to the five parameters already mentioned, these workers found that the duration of chest pain symptoms, other risk factors (blood pressure,

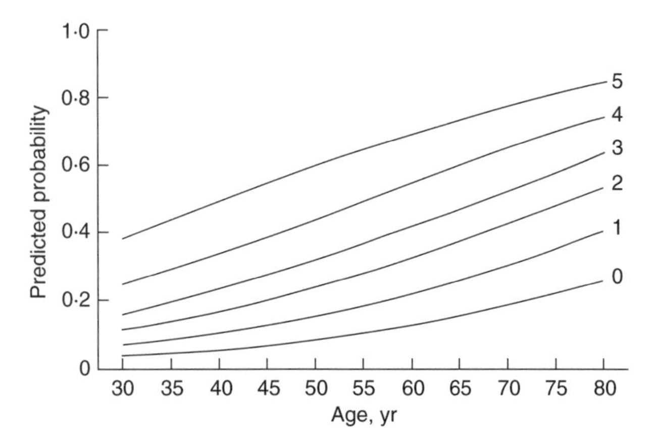

Figure 3.2 Nomogram showing the probability of severe (three vessel or left main) coronary artery disease based on a 5 point score. One point is awarded for each of the following variables – male gender, typical angina, history, and electrocardiographic evidence of MI, diabetes, and use of insulin. Each curve shows the probability of severe coronary disease as a function of age. (From Hubbard *et al*,[8] with permission.)

hyperlipidemia, and smoking), a carotid bruit, and chest pain frequency were also important determinants of the likelihood of severe CAD. However, the magnitude of their additional effect was modest.

Prediction of patient outcome

The ability of clinical assessment to predict patient outcome has been demonstrated in numerous previous studies. The largest and most important of these came from the Duke University databank[10] and the Coronary Artery Surgical Study Registry.[11] Many of the same parameters that predict the presence of disease and the presence of severe disease are also associated with adverse patient outcome. Age, gender, chest pain description, and previous myocardial infarction all have independent value in predicting patient outcome. In addition, history and physical examination evidence for congestive heart failure, history and physical examination evidence of vascular disease, unstable chest pain characteristics, and other ECG findings, such as ST-T wave changes, left bundle branch block, and intraventricular conduction delay, all have prognostic value. It is not generally appreciated how well clinical parameters perform in this regard. The Duke group reported that 37% of the patients undergoing stress testing at their institution had a predicted average annual mortality of 1% or less over the next 3 years, on the basis of clinical assessment.[11]

Several studies have shown that a normal resting ECG, and the absence of a history of prior infarction, predict a normal ejection fraction with 90% confidence,[12,13] and therefore a favorable prognosis.[14–16]

Approaches to the assessment of incremental value

Once the information available from clinical assessment (and other tests already performed) has been considered, there are a variety of conceptual and statistical approaches that can be employed to assess the incremental value of the test in question. This section will present examples of three such approaches.

Diagnosis of CAD

The application of multiple different stress tests for the diagnosis of coronary artery disease has been extensively studied. The most common approach used in this setting to demonstrate the incremental value of a new test employs Bayes' theorem.[17] This theorem indicates that the likelihood of disease following testing (post-test probability) can be calculated from the test characteristics (sensitivity and specificity) and the pretest probability. This calculated post-test probability is often plotted graphically as a function of pretest probability (Figure 3.3).

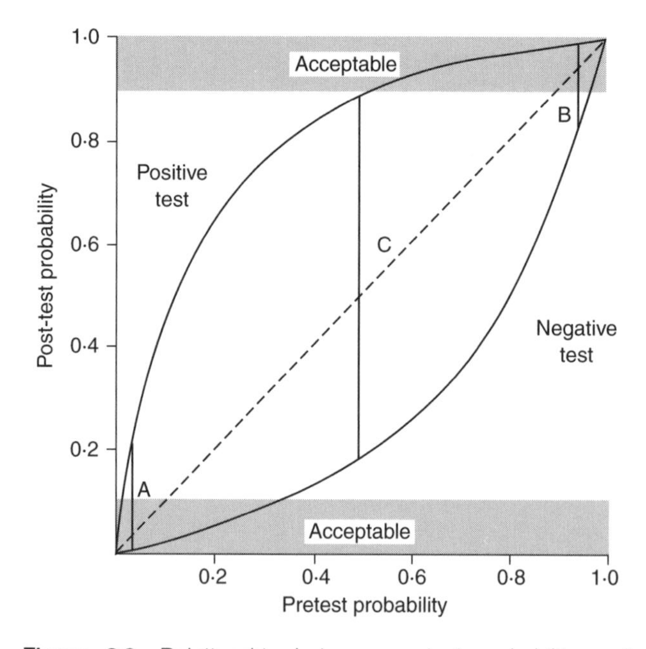

Figure 3.3 Relationship between pretest probability and post-test probability. The solid curves for positive and negative tests are plotted for a test with 80% sensitivity and a 90% specificity. Post-test probabilities that are acceptable for diagnosis (90% and 10%) are shown in the shaded zones. Line A represents a patient with a very low pretest probability; line B, a patient with a high pretest probability; line C, a patient with an intermediate probability. (Modified from Berman DS, Garcia EV, Maddahi J. Thallium-201 scintigraphy in the detection and evaluation of coronary artery disease. In: Berman DS, Mason DT, eds. *Clinical nuclear cardiology*. New York: Grune and Stratton, 1981, with permission.)

In Figure 3.3, the pretest probability is shown on the *X*-axis and the post-test probability is shown on the *Y*-axis. The dotted line represents the line of identity. The vertical distance from this line to the upper solid curve represents the increase in the probability of disease as a result of positive test. In analogous fashion, the vertical distance from this dotted line to the lower solid curve represents the decrease in probability as a result of a negative test. The solid vertical lines describe three different clinical situations.

Line A represents a patient with a very low pretest probability, such as a 40 year old woman with non-anginal pain. A negative test changes probability very little. A positive test increases probability somewhat, but the post-test probability remains well under 50%, and the test is most likely a "false positive".

Line B represents a patient with a high pretest probability of disease, such as a 65 year old man with typical angina. A positive test will increase the probability only slightly. A negative test will decrease the probability of disease somewhat, but the post-test probability remains substantially greater than 50%, so that the test is most likely a "false negative".

The final situation (line C) represents a patient with an intermediate probability of disease, such as a 50 year old male with atypical angina. A positive test in such a patient would increase the probability of disease substantially to near 90%. On the other hand a negative test would decrease the probability of disease substantially to approximately 18%.

Thus, it is evident that the incremental value of diagnostic testing is greater in patients with an intermediate probability of disease, a principle that is broadly recognized.[17]

However, it is also recognized that this kind of analysis has a number of limitations. The single curves for positive and negative tests do not take into account the degree of test abnormality. The test results are therefore better displayed for a whole range of values for a parameter that helps distinguish normal from abnormal. The best known example of this would be the magnitude of ST segment depression on treadmill exercise testing.[18] In addition, multiple other parameters are reported during a treadmill exercise test, which help to distinguish severely abnormal tests from only mildly abnormal tests.[19] Ideally, all of these parameters would be incorporated into a single "score" and a series of curves would be plotted.

Next, construction of such curves relies on the premise that the sensitivity of tests will be identical for any population of patients with disease regardless of disease prevalence. This assumption is usually invalid. As demonstrated in the previous section, those parameters which help to identify the presence of disease also help to identify the presence of severe disease. In general, the sensitivity of most tests is greater in patients with more severe disease. It is therefore quickly evident that sensitivity would be expected to vary with the prevalence of disease. This point has been demonstrated by several investigators,[20] and provides justification for the use of logistic regression analysis for diagnostic purposes.[21] Despite these limitations, bayesian analysis serves as a useful framework for understanding the potential incremental value of diagnostic tests.

Post-test referral bias, also known as work up bias or verification bias, occurs whenever the results of the test in question influence the subsequent performance of the "reference" test (sometimes referred to as the "gold standard"). This bias has been recognized for more than 20 years.[22] An early survey of the literature on exercise testing showed that only 2 of 33 studies avoided this bias.[23] The recognition of the importance of this phenomenon was emphasized in a landmark paper in 1983, which described the "declining specificity" of radionuclide angiography as a result of this bias.[24] More than 10 years ago, a monograph from the Institute of Medicine emphasized this well established concept.[25] The key question to ascertain whether postreferral bias is present is "did the results of the test being evaluated influence the decision to perform reference standard?".[26]

Although this bias potentially occurs for any diagnostic test, it is particularly important for non-invasive diagnostic tests for CAD. Patients with positive non-invasive tests are often referred to coronary angiography (the "reference" test). In contrast, patients with negative tests are often sent home without coronary angiography. The effects of this preferential referral to coronary angiography are to markedly decrease the observed specificity of the test in question and modestly increase its sensitivity.

The clearest solution to the problem of post-test referral bias is to avoid it completely by studying patients in whom the decision to proceed with the "reference" test is made before the performance of the diagnostic test in question.[25] For the diagnosis of CAD, this standard is incredibly difficult and rarely achieved. A more feasible alternative is the mathematical correction of sensitivity and specificity for post-test referral bias using one of two published formulae and information about all of the patients who were studied using the diagnostic test in question and did not proceed with coronary angiography.[27,28] There are a number of published studies demonstrating the effect of these corrections on the observed test performance for exercise electrocardiographic testing,[29] exercise echocardiography,[30] and exercise Single Photon Computed Tomography (SPECT) perfusion imaging.[31] Correction for referral bias markedly increases the specificity and modestly decreases the sensitivity of these tests. As a result, the predictive value of a positive test is improved, but the predictive value of a negative test decreases. It is generally difficult to confirm the validity of these corrections. However, a carefully designed prospective study of exercise echocardiography in women has now reported sensitivity and specificity values that are very close to those reported after correction for referral bias.[32]

Post-test referral bias has numerous important implications for the interpretation of the diagnostic literature.[32] Many of the reported sensitivity and specificity values are very likely to be erroneous.[32] Widespread misconceptions exist regarding gender differences in test performance. The post-test probability of CAD is higher for either a positive or negative test than that which would be calculated from Bayes' theorem using the reported values of sensitivity and specificity.[31]

Non-invasive screening for severe CAD

The incremental value of testing for the diagnosis of severe CAD has been studied using both bayesian analysis and logistic regression analysis. When the latter analysis is conducted properly, all of the previously discussed clinical parameters that are associated with severe coronary disease are incorporated into a model that is used to predict the probability of severe CAD. The output of such a model is a probability that ranges between 0 and 1. It is critically important that these candidate variables be "forced" into the model, even if they are statistically insignificant in the population under study. Most study populations are too small to have adequate power to detect the true significance of these variables, which has been demonstrated in very large subsets. For example, age should always be forced into such models, even if it does not appear to be significant in the particular population in question, because there is abundant evidence that it should always be considered (and indeed usually is by clinicians).

Using this approach, a second model should then be constructed which includes all of the clinical parameters, as well as pertinent new parameters from the test in question. If these parameters have statistical significance independent of the clinical parameters, the test has incremental value. This approach is demonstrated in Table 3.2, which shows the improvement in the logistic regression model for severe CAD reported by Christian *et al*,[16] when the exercise test was added to clinical parameters, and when thallium imaging parameters were added to clinical and exercise parameters. An alternative approach is to construct the receiver operating characteristic (ROC) curves, which display sensitivity and specificity as a function of the predicted probability of severe disease (the output of a logistic regression model). The area under the ROC curve can then be compared between the model that incorporates clinical parameters,

Table 3.2 Logistic regression multivariate analysis: prediction of three vessel or left main (coronary artery) disease

Model	Direction	Odds ratio (95% CI)	*P* value
Clinical			
Diabetes mellitus	Present	2·0 (1·3–3·1)	0·001
Typical angina	Present	2·3 (1·4–3·9)	0·001
Sex	Male	3·2 (1·4–4·0)	0·007
Age[a]	Older	1·4 (1·1–1·9)	0·01
$\chi^2 = 31{\cdot}3$			
Clinical and exercise			
Diabetes mellitus	Present	1·9 (1·2–3·0)	0·005
Typical angina	Present	1·9 (1·1–3·3)	0·02
Sex	Male	2·3 (0·9–5·3)	0·07
Age[a]	Older	1·2 (0·9–1·7)	0·16
Magnitude of ST depression	More	1·5 (1·3–1·8)	<0·001
Peak heart rate × peak systolic blood pressure[b]	Lower	0·9 (0·86–0·95)	<0·001
$\chi^2 = 65{\cdot}0$			
Clinical, exercise, and thallium-201			
Diabetes mellitus	Present	1·9 (1·2–3·0)	0·004
Typical angina	Present	1·8 (1·1–3·2)	0·03
Sex	Male	2·2 (0·9–5·3)	0·07
Age[a]	Older	1·2 (0·9–1·7)	0·17
Peak heart rate × peak systolic blood pressure[b]	Lower	0·9 (0·86–0·95)	<0·001
Magnitude of ST depression	More	1·4 (1·2–1·7)	0·001
Global T1-201 score (delayed – after exercise)	Higher	1·1 (1·0–1·1)	0.02
$\chi^2 = 70{\cdot}4$			

[a] Increments of 10 years (each 10-year increase in age increases the odds of severe disease 1·4-fold).
[b] Increments of 1000 units.
From Christian TF *et al*,[16] with permission

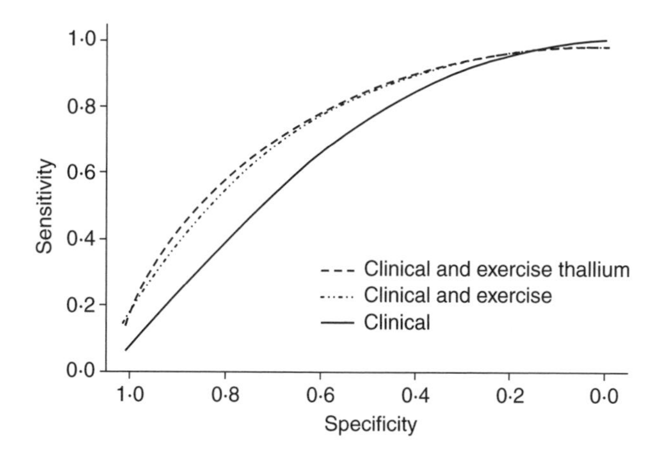

Figure 3.4 Receiver operator characteristic curves for three logistic regression multivariate models for the prediction of severe coronary disease. (From Christian *et al*,[16] with permission.)

and the model that incorporates clinical parameters and the new test parameters. Methods are available for determining the statistical significance of changes in the area under these two ROC curves.[33] An example of this approach is shown in Figure 3.4, taken from Christian *et al*[16] The clinical significance of these differences in the models (assessed by either χ^2 analysis or ROC curves) is discussed later.

Prediction of patient outcome

The demonstration of incremental prognostic value for diagnostic tests is obviously extremely important for clinical decision making. It requires strict adherence to the rigorous standards that were outlined previously. In general, very few of the published studies demonstrating prognostic value of diagnostic tests meet the strict criteria necessary to demonstrate *incremental* prognostic value for these tests. The statistical model most often used for this purpose is a linear proportional hazards, or Cox, model.[34] When strictly applied, all the previous information available to the clinician, either from clinical assessment or previous testing, should be incorporated into a linear proportional hazards model that predicts time to an event. Once again, parameters that have been clearly demonstrated in larger populations to be significant must be "forced" into such models to make sure that their contribution is not neglected. The events in question should preferably be hard end points such as death and myocardial infarction. As previously mentioned, unstable angina and the need for revascularization are alternative end points that are often included to enhance statistical power, but these have major limitations.

One of the best examples of a rigorously constructed analysis demonstrating incremental prognostic value was published by Pollock *et al* in 1992.[35] They tested the association between various combinations of variables, and time to death or myocardial infarction, in a linear proportional hazards model using the χ^2 statistic. Clinical and exercise variables were significantly better than clinical variables alone. Similarly, a model that added thallium redistribution to clinical and exercise variables was significantly better than the combination of clinical and exercise variables.

Another example of such a rigorous analysis was that reported by Christian *et al*[6] in patients with a normal resting electrocardiogram. Using a similar approach, these investigators reported that a model adding thallium variables to clinical and exercise variables did not add significantly to the model using clinical and exercise variables. Thus, in the subset of patients with a normal resting ECG, Christian *et al*[16] were unable to confirm the findings of Pollock *et al*[24]

Clinical significance and cost effectiveness

Even when statistically significant incremental value has been demonstrated for a diagnostic test using appropriate rigorous methodology, the clinical significance of the findings must be equally rigorously examined. The two fundamental issues that should be addressed are the actual impact of this incremental value on clinical decision making and, where possible, cost effectiveness. The principles of decision analysis pertinent to the first criterion will be presented in much greater detail in Chapter 7. The available published data on diagnostic testing in coronary disease that will be presented here use only rudimentary concepts with respect to decision analysis. Formal cost analysis also requires understanding of a much greater body of published knowledge, which will not be presented here. The examples presented will again be very rudimentary, but demonstrate the principle.

Diagnosis of CAD

The clinical significance of diagnostic testing can best be understood in terms of decision making thresholds. From the standpoint of diagnosis, a test will be useful primarily if it moves a significant number of patients from an "uncertain" pretest probability to an "acceptably certain" post-test probability. The exact criteria, or threshold, to be used in these classifications are clearly a matter of judgment; many investigators have chosen post-test probabilities of less than 10% and greater than 90% as criteria for definitive diagnosis.[36] Thus, non-invasive testing will be useful for diagnosis if it moves a reasonable number of patients into the shaded zone shown in Figure 3.3.

Although treadmill testing has clear incremental value for diagnosis, particularly in patients with intermediate pretest probability, as discussed earlier, its ability to move patients across such thresholds of probability appears to be very limited. Goldman *et al*[37] examined the ability of treadmill

Table 3.3 Effect of treadmill exercise test results in moving patients across various diagnostic thresholds

Threshold probability	Patients moved across (*n*)	Correctly moved	Incorrectly moved	Net increase in diagnoses (correct-incorrect)
0·10	8	6	2	4
0·90	53	33	20	13
Either 0·10 or 0·90	61	39	22	17 (5%)

From Goldman *et al*,[37] by permission of the American Heart Association, Inc.

exercise variables to classify 329 patients with CAD. Their results are summarized in Table 3.3. The pretest model was very powerful, as it classified 84% of the patients correctly. Table 3.3 shows the number of additional patients classified correctly for given thresholds of probability. For example, if 10% was considered an acceptable threshold to "rule out" CAD, eight of 324 patients were moved across this threshold, but only six were moved correctly. Similarly, for a 90% threshold to "rule in" CAD, 53 patients were moved across this threshold but only 33 were moved across correctly. As a result, the net total number of patients who were correctly moved into the diagnostic zone in Figure 3.3 was only 17, or 5% of the patient population. Thus, the clinical significance of the incremental value provided by the treadmill test appears to be very limited.

Similar rigorous analyses have been published for radionuclide angiography.[38] The results of one of these are displayed in Figure 3.5. The study group excluded men with typical angina over the age of 40 in order to eliminate most patients with a high pretest probability. Logistic regression models developed on a retrospective population were applied prospectively to a group of 76 patients. As demonstrated in Figure 3.5, eight (11%) of the 76 patients could be classified with 90% certainty on the basis of clinical variables alone. Following radionuclide angiography, 24 patients (32%) could be classified directly. Thus, the incremental value of exercise radionuclide angiography in moving patients across clinically meaningful decision thresholds appeared to be much greater than for the treadmill exercise test, as 21% of the patients were correctly classified by the radionuclide angiogram.

Similar findings have been reported for planar thallium imaging.[39,40] Unfortunately, no rigorous analyses are available for either SPECT imaging or sestamibi imaging, primarily because post-test selection bias has greatly limited the feasibility of such studies in the current era.

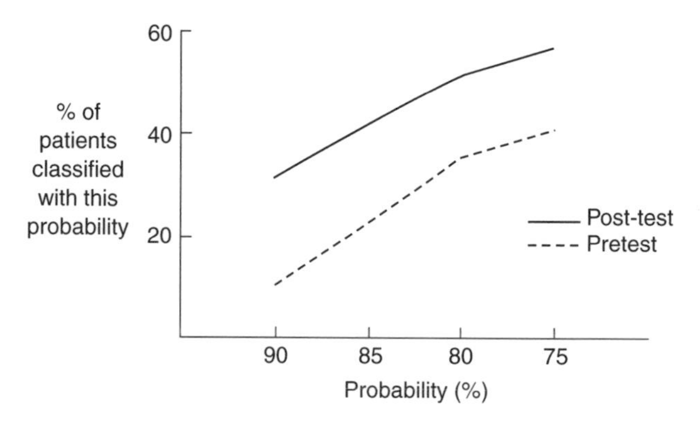

Figure 3.5 Percentage of patients classified with a given probability of coronary disease before and after exercise radionuclide angiography. The prospective study group of 76 patients excluded males of 40 years or older with typical angina. (From Gibbons *et al*,[38] with permission.)

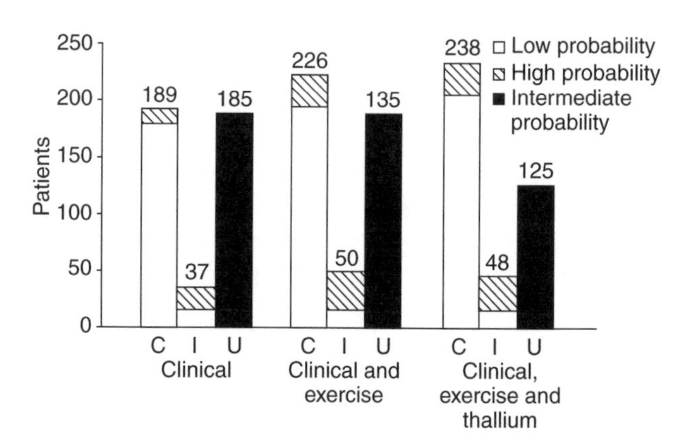

Figure 3.6 Correct (C), incorrect (I), and uncertain (U) classification of patients with three vessel or left main coronary artery disease by the use of logistic regression multivariate models. Low, intermediate, and high probability defined using: clinical variables only; clinical and exercise variables; clinical, exercise, and thallium-201 variables. (From Christian *et al*,[16] with permission.)

Non-invasive screening for severe CAD

The same threshold approach has been applied to the non-invasive identification of severe CAD. Here the ability of tests to move patients across somewhat different thresholds of probability, as assessed by logistic regression models, has been tested. Christian *et al*[16] defined a low-probability group for severe CAD as <0·15, a high-risk group as >0·35, and an intermediate group as 0·15–0·35. These thresholds were chosen to correspond to earlier work from Duke University reporting on the utility of the early positive treadmill test.[41] Figure 3.6 shows the results that were obtained using this approach. Using clinical parameters alone, 189 patients (46% of the study group) were correctly classified as low or high probability. Thirty-seven patients (9%) were incorrectly classified as low or high probability. The remaining 185 patients (45% of the study group) had an intermediate probability, and were therefore in an uncertain category. The addition of exercise parameters correctly classified an additional 37 patients at the expense of 13 additional incorrect classifications, for a net of 24 additional correct classifications (6% of the study group). The addition of thallium parameters led to 12 additional correct classifications, and two fewer incorrect classifications for a net increase of 14 correct classifications (3% of the study group). These workers then used Medicare reimbursement figures to calculate the cost per additional correct classification. For exercise testing, the cost per additional correct patient classification was $1524. For thallium scintigraphy, the cost was $20 550 per additional correct classification.

Thus, this analysis demonstrated that the clinical impact was modest, and the cost was high, when thallium imaging was used in patients with a normal resting ECG to try to identify patients non-invasively with severe CAD. Although thallium scintigraphy clearly had statistically significant incremental value, it did not appear to be cost effective for this purpose.

Prediction of patient outcome

The issues of clinical significance and cost effectiveness are particularly pertinent to the application of diagnostic tests for the prediction of the patient outcome. These applications often involve relatively low-risk patient groups with few subsequent events. Tests applied to the entire population may identify a subset of patients who are at considerably increased risk.[42,43] These results will be highly statistically significant, and generate very impressive *P* values and risk ratios. However, it must be recognized that the absolute rate of events often remains too low in the high-risk patient subgroup to be clinically meaningful, and the cost of this identification is often therefore prohibitive when viewed on a per event basis.

This concept was nicely demonstrated in a study by Berman *et al*[44] on patients with a low clinical likelihood of CAD studied by SPECT sestamibi. During 20 months of follow up, only patients with an abnormal sestamibi study suffered death or myocardial infarction. This difference was statistically highly significant ($P = 0 \cdot 007$). However, this increment in prognostic value was clearly not cost effective, as noted by the authors. Although the cost analysis by the authors was quite detailed, the cost ineffectiveness of this approach is readily apparent with very simple analysis. The 107 patients in the high-risk group suffered only three events during 20 months of follow up. In order to identify the high-risk group, testing was required of 548 patients. Using a Medicare reimbursement figure of $700 per test,[16] more than $383 000 of testing would be required to identify the high-risk cohort. The cost of testing alone would therefore exceed $127 000 per possible event prevented. This simple analysis ignores the additional costs that would accrue from the subsequent cardiac catheterizations and coronary revascularizations that would be necessary in the high-risk group in order to attempt to prevent the three events. (There is obviously no certainty that the three events could actually be prevented by revascularization.)

Similar analyses have been published for screening in asymptomatic individuals. As a general principle, it should be recognized that non-invasive testing for the assessment of prognosis is far less cost effective in subsets of patients at intrinsically low risk.

Conclusion

Clinicians should recognize that an evidence-based approach to the evaluation of the incremental value of diagnostic tests is not simple or straightforward. Unfortunately, it is far easier for both clinicians and investigators to use simple, less rigorous, approaches that appear to demonstrate important incremental value for each new diagnostic test. Although convenient, such approaches lead to incorrect conclusions, and generally overestimate the added value of each new testing modality. The examples presented in this chapter should provide a framework for thinking clinicians to evaluate better new publications on new diagnostic tests. However difficult these analyses may be, and however disappointing the results, the escalating costs of healthcare demand an approach of rigorous methodology and thoughtful analysis to make certain that the *incremental* value of a diagnostic test is not only statistically significant, but clinically significant and cost effective.

References

1. Diamond G. Penny wise. *Am J Cardiol* 1988;**62**:806–8.
2. Bobbio M, Pollock BH, Cohen I, Diamond GA. Comparative accuracy of clinical tests for diagnosis and prognosis of coronary artery disease. *Am J Cardiol* 1988;**62**:896–900.
3. Ladenheim ML, Kotler TS, Pollock BH, Berman DS, Diamond GA. Incremental prognostic power of clinical history, exercise electrocardiography and myocardial perfusion scintigraphy in suspected coronary artery disease. *Am J Cardiol* 1987;**59**: 270–7.
4. Diamond GA, Forrester JS. Analysis of probability as an aid in the clinical diagnosis of coronary artery disease. *N Engl J Med* 1979;**300**:1350–8.
5. Diamond GA. Letter: a clinical relevant classification of chest discomfort. *J Am Coll Cardiol* 1983;**1**:574–5.

6.Pryor DB, Harrell FE Jr, Lee KL, Califf RM, Rosati RA. Estimating the likelihood of significant coronary artery disease. *Am J Med* 1983;**75**:771–80.
7.Weiner DA, McCabe CH, Ryan TJ. Identification of patients with left main and three vessel coronary disease with clinical and exercise test variables. *Am J Cardiol* 1980;**46**:21–7.
8.Hubbard BL, Gibbons RJ, Lapeyre AC, Zinsmeister AR, Clements IP. Identification of severe coronary artery disease using simple clinical parameters. *Arch Intern Med* 1992;**152**: 309–12.
9.Pryor DB, Shaw L, Harrell FE Jr *et al.* Estimating the likelihood of severe coronary artery disease. *Am J Med* 1991;**90**: 553–62.
10.Pryor DB, Shaw L, McCants CB *et al.* Value of the history and physical in identifying patients at increased risk for coronary artery disease. *Ann Intern Med* 1993;**118**:81–90.
11.Weiner DA, Ryan TJ, McCabe CH *et al.* The role of exercise testing in identifying patients with improved survival after coronary artery bypass surgery. *J Am Coll Cardiol* 1986;**8**: 741–8.
12.O'Keefe JH Jr, Zinsmeister AR, Gibbons RJ. Value of electrocardiographic findings in predicting rest left ventricular function in patients with chest pain and suspected coronary artery disease. *Am J Med* 1989;**86**:658–62.
13.Rihal CS, Davis KB, Kennedy JW, Gersh BJ. The utility of clinical, electrocardiographic, and roentgenographic variables in the prediction of left ventricular function. *Am J Cardiol* 1995;**75**:220–3.
14.Connolly DC, Elveback LR, Oxman HA. Coronary heart disease in residents of Rochester, Minnesota. IV. Prognostic value of the resting electrocardiogram at the time of initial diagnosis of angina pectoris. *Mayo Clin Proc* 1984;**59**:247–50.
15.Gibbons RJ, Zinsmeister AR, Miller TD, Clements IP. Supine exercise electrocardiography compared with exercise radionuclide angiography in noninvasive identification of severe coronary artery disease. *Ann Intern Med* 1990;**112**:743–9.
16.Christian TF, Miller TD, Bailey KR, Gibbons RJ. Exercise tomographic thallium-201 imaging in patients with severe coronary artery disease and normal electrocardiogram. *Ann Intern Med* 1994;**121**:825–32.
17.Epstein SE. Implications of probability analysis on the strategy used for noninvasive detection of coronary artery disease. *Am J Cardiol* 1980;**46**:491–9.
18.Rifkin RD, Hood WB Jr. Bayesian analysis of electrocardiographic exercise stress testing. *N Engl J Med* 1977;**297**: 681–6.
19.Cohn K, Kamm B, Feteih N, Brand R, Goldschlager N. Use of treadmill score to quantify ischemic response and predict extent of coronary disease. *Circulation* 1979;**59**:286–96.
20.Currie PJ, Kelly MJ, Harper RW *et al.* Incremental value of clinical assessment, supine exercise electrocardiography, and biplane exercise radionuclide ventriculography in the prediction of coronary artery disease in men with chest pain. *Am J Cardiol* 1983;**52**:927–35.
21.Morise AP, Detrano R, Bobbio M, Diamond GA. Development and validation of a logistic regression-derived algorithm for estimating the incremental probability of coronary artery disease before and after exercise testing. *J Am Coll Cardiol* 1992; **20**:1187–96.
22.Ransohoff DF, Feinstein AR. Problems of spectrum and bias in evaluating the efficacy of diagnostic tests. *N Engl J Med* 1978; **299**:926–30.
23.Philbrick JT, Horwitz RI, Feinstein AR. Methodologic problems of exercise testing for coronary artery disease: groups, analysis and bias. *Am J Cardiol* 1980;**46**:807–12.
24.Rozanski A, Diamond GA, Berman D, Forrester JS, Morris D, Swan HJC. The declining specificity of exercise radionuclide ventriculography. *N Engl J Med* 1983; **309**:518–22.
25.Council on Health Care Technology, Institute of Medicine. *Assessment of diagnostic technology in health care.* Washington, DC: National Academy Press,1989.
26.Jaeschke R, Guyatt G, Sackett DL. Users' guides to the medical literature. *JAMA* 1994; **271**:389–91.
27.Diamond GA. An alternative factor affecting sensitivity and specificity of exercise electrocardiology (editorial). *Am J Cardiol* 1986; **57**:1175–80.
28.Begg CB, Greenes RA. Assessment of diagnostic tests when disease verification is subject to selection bias. *Biometrics* 1983;**39**:207–15.
29.Morise AP, Diamond GA. Comparison of the sensitivity and specificity of exercise electrocardiography in biased and unbiased populations of men and women. *Am Heart J* 1995; **130**:741–7.
30.Roger VL, Pellikka PA, Bell MR, Chow CWH, Bailey KR, Seward JB. Sex and test verification bias: Impact on the Diagnostic Value of Exercise Echocardiology. *Circulation* 1997; **95**:405–10.
31.Miller TD, Hodge DO, Christian TF, Milavetz JJ, Bailey KR, Gibbons RJ. Effects on adjustment for referral bias on the sensitivity of specificity of single photon emission computed tomography for the diagnosis of coronary artery disease. *Am J Med* 2002;**112**:290–7.
32.Gibbons RJ, Chatterjee K, Daley J, *et al.* ACC/AHA/ACP-ASIM guidelines for the management of patients with chronic stable angina: a report of the American College of Cardiology/ American Heart Association Task Force on Practice Guidelines (Committee on the Management of Patients With Chronic Stable Angina). *J Am Coll Cardiol* 1999;**33**:2092–7.
33.Wieand S, Gail M, James K, James B. A family of nonparametric statistics for comparing diagnostic tests with paired or unpaired data. *Biometrika* 1989;**76**:585–92.
34.Cox DR. Regression models and life tables. *J R Stat Soc B* 1972;**34**:197–220.
35.Pollock SG, Abbott RD, Boucher CA, Beller GA, Kaul S. Independent and incremental prognostic value of tests performed in hierarchical order to evaluate patients with suspected coronary artery disease. Validation of models based on these tests. *Circulation* 1992;**85**:237–48.
36.Diamond GA, Forrester JS, Hirsch M *et al.* Application of conditional probability analysis to the clinical diagnosis of coronary artery disease. *J Clin Invest* 1980;**65**:1210–21.
37.Goldman L, Cook EF, Mitchell N *et al.* Incremental value of the exercise test for diagnosing the presence or absence of coronary artery disease. *Circulation* 1982;**66**:945–53.
38.Gibbons RJ, Lee KL, Pryor DB *et al.* The use of radionuclide angiography in the diagnosis of coronary artery disease: a logistic regression analysis. *Circulation* 1983;**68**:740–6.
39.Detrano R, Yiannikas J, Salcedo EE *et al.* Bayesian probability analysis: a prospective demonstration of its clinical utility in diagnosing coronary disease. *Circulation* 1984;**69**: 541–7.

40.Melin JA, Wijns W, Vanbutsele RJ *et al.* Alternative diagnostic strategies for coronary artery disease in women: demonstration of the usefulness and efficiency of probability analysis. *Circulation* 1985;**71**:535–42.
41.McNeer JF, Margolis JR, Lee KL *et al.* The role of the exercise test in the evaluation of patients for ischemic heart disease. *Circulation* 1978;**57**:64–70.
42.Rautaharju PM, Prineas RJ, Eifler WJ *et al.* Prognostic value of exercise electrocardiogram in men at high risk of future coronary heart disease: multiple risk factor intervention trial experience. *J Am Coll Cardiol* 1986;**8**:1–10.
43.Giagnoni E, Secchi MB, Wu SC *et al.* Prognostic value of exercise EKG testing in asymptomatic normotensive subjects: a prospective matched study. *N Engl J Med* 1983;**309**: 1085–9.
44.Berman DS, Hachamovitch R, Hosen K *et al.* Incremental value of prognostic testing in patients with known or suspected ischemic heart disease: a basis for optimal utilization of exercise technetium-99 m sestamibi myocardial perfusion single-photon emission computed tomography. *J Am Coll Cardiol* 1995;**26**:639–47.

4 Clinical trials and meta-analysis

Colin Baigent

Introduction

Although large effects on survival arising from certain treatments may occasionally be obvious from simple observation (as, for example, when cardioversion for ventricular fibrillation avoids otherwise certain death), the vast majority of interventions have only moderate effects on major outcomes and hence are impossible to evaluate without careful study. Enthusiasm for the biologic foundations of a particular therapeutic approach often leads to exaggerated hopes for the effects of treatment on major clinical outcomes. These hopes may be based on dramatic laboratory measures of efficacy, or on the types of surrogate outcome that are commonly studied before drugs go into Phase III or IV studies: for example, a drug may almost completely prevent experimental ischemia progressing to infarction, or practically abolish experimental thrombosis. However, these large effects on surrogate end points very rarely translate into large effects on major clinical outcomes: the overwhelming message from two decades of clinical trials in cardiology is that the net effects of most treatments are typically moderate in size.* This chapter explains why large-scale randomized evidence, either in a single "mega-trial" or in a meta-analysis of similar trials, is generally an absolute requirement if such moderate effects on major outcomes are to be characterized reliably.

It is important to appreciate that progress in cardiologic practice, and in the prevention of cardiovascular disease, has been and remains dependent on the availability of large-scale randomized trials and appropriately large-scale meta-analyses of such trials. In the management of acute myocardial infarction (MI), for example, these methods have helped to demonstrate that fibrinolytic therapy,[1–3] aspirin,[1,3,4] angiotensin-converting-enzyme (ACE) inhibitors[5–7] and β-blockers[8] all produce net benefits which, although individually moderate in size, have together produced a substantial improvement in the prognosis of acute MI. Similarly, the demonstration that ACE inhibitors produce moderate reductions in the risk of death and in the rates of hospitalization for worsening heart failure,[9] and that the addition of digoxin further reduces the need for recurrent hospitalization,[10] has improved the prognosis of congestive heart failure.

Clinical trials: minimizing biases and random errors

Any clinical study whose main objective is to assess moderate treatment effects must ensure that any biases and any random errors that are inherent in its design are both substantially smaller than the effect to be measured.[11,12] Biases in the assessment of treatment can be produced by differences in factors other than the treatment under consideration. Observational (that is non-randomized) studies in which the outcome is compared between individuals who received the treatment of interest and those who did not, can be subject to large biases.[13] Instead, the guaranteed avoidance of biases requires the proper randomized allocation of treatment and appropriate statistical analysis, with no unduly data-dependent emphasis on specific subsets of the overall evidence (Table 4.1).[12]

Avoidance of moderate biases

Proper randomization

The fundamental reason for random allocation of treatment in clinical trials is to maximize the likelihood that each type of patient will have been allocated in similar proportions to the different treatment strategies being investigated.[14] Proper randomization requires that trial procedures are organized in a way that ensures that the decision to enter a patient is made irreversibly and without knowledge of the trial treatment to which a patient will be allocated. In situations where the next treatment allocation can be deduced by those entering patients, decisions about whether to enter a

* For rare adverse effects, however, there may be large proportional differences between one treatment and another, or between treatment and control. For example, some non-steroidal anti-inflammatory drugs may substantially increase the risk of gastrointestinal bleeding. Rare adverse effects with extreme relative risks can often be recognized reliably by careful clinical observation, or by other non-randomized methods, and such relative risks are sometimes best quantified in case–control or cohort studies.

Table 4.1 Requirements for reliable assessment of MODERATE treatment effects[11,12]

1. *Negligible biases*
   (that is guaranteed avoidance of MODERATE biases)
   - Proper RANDOMIZATION (non-randomized methods cannot guarantee the avoidance of moderate biases)
   - Analysis by ALLOCATED treatments (that is an "intention to treat" analysis)
   - Chief emphasis on OVERALL results (with no unduly data-derived subgroup analysis)
   - Systematic META-ANALYSIS of all the relevant randomized trials (with no unduly data-dependent emphasis on the results from particular studies)
2. *Small random errors*
   (that is guaranteed avoidance of MODERATE random errors)
   - LARGE NUMBERS (with minimal data collection as detailed statistical analyses of masses of data on prognostic features generally add little to the effective size of a trial)
   - Systematic META-ANALYSIS of all the relevant randomized trials

particular patient may be affected, and those allocated one treatment might then differ systematically from those allocated another.[15] In the Captopril Prevention Project (CAPPP) trial,[16] for example, envelopes containing the antihypertensive treatment allocation could be opened before patients were irreversibly entered into the study. Highly significant differences in pre-entry blood pressure between the treatment groups, which were too large to have been due to chance, may well have been the result of this design weakness.[17]

Intention to treat analysis

Even when studies have been properly randomized and well conducted, moderate biases can still be introduced by inappropriate analysis or interpretation. One well recognized circumstance is when patients are excluded after randomization, particularly when the prognosis of the excluded patients in one treatment group differs from that in the other (such as might occur, for example, if non-compliers were excluded after randomization). This point is well illustrated by the Coronary Drug Project, which compared clofibrate versus placebo among around 5000 patients with a history of coronary heart disease. In this study, patients who took at least 80% of their allocated clofibrate ("good" compliers) had substantially lower 5 year mortality than "poor" compliers who did not (15·0% *v* 24·6% respectively; $P = 0{\cdot}0001$). However, there was a similar difference in outcome between "good" and "poor" compliers in the placebo group (15·1% *v* 28·3%, respectively; $P < 0{\cdot}00001$), suggesting that "good" and "poor" compliers were prognostically different even after allowing for any benefits of actually taking clofibrate.[18] If there is really no difference in outcome between two treatments, then the least biased assessment of the treatment effect is that which compares all those allocated to one treatment versus all those allocated to the other (that is an "intention to treat" analysis), irrespective of what treatment they actually received.[19]

Because some degree of non-compliance with allocated treatments is unavoidable in randomized trials, intention to treat analyses will obviously underestimate the effects produced by full compliance. However, "on treatment" analyses, which compare effects among compliant patients with those in non-compliant patients, are potentially biased, and it is more appropriate to calculate an "adjustment" based on the level of compliance and then to apply this to the estimate of the treatment effect provided by the intention to treat comparison.[20] For example, in a meta-analysis of the randomized trials of prolonged use of antiplatelet therapy among patients with occlusive vascular disease, the average compliance 1 year after treatment allocation seemed to be around 80%.[4] Application of this estimate of compliance to the proportional reduction of about 30% in non-fatal MI and stroke estimated from intention to treat analyses of these trials suggests that full compliance with antiplatelet therapy produces reductions in risk of about 35–40%.

Dangers of data-dependent emphasis on particular results

In the medical literature a particularly important source of bias is unduly data-dependent emphasis on particular trials or on particular subgroups of patients. Such emphasis is often entirely inadvertent, arising from a perfectly reasonable desire to understand the randomized trial results in terms of who to treat, which treatments to prefer, or disease mechanisms. However, whatever its origins, selective emphasis on particular parts of the evidence can often lead to seriously misleading conclusions. This is because the identification of categories of patients for whom treatment is particularly effective (or ineffective) requires surprisingly large quantities of data. Even if the real sizes of the treatment effects do vary substantially among subgroups of patients, subgroup analyses are so statistically insensitive that they may well fail to demonstrate these differences. On the other hand, if the real proportional risk reductions are about the same for everybody, subgroup analyses can vary so widely just by the play of chance that the results in selected subgroups may be exaggerated. Even when highly significant "interactions" are found, they may be a poor guide to the sizes (or even the directions) of any genuine differences, as the more extreme such results may still owe more to chance than to reality. This is particularly the case when such interactions have emerged after an overzealous examination of multiple subgroups. For example, in the large Second International Study of Infarct Survival (ISIS-2), the 1 month survival advantage produced by aspirin was particularly clear (804 vascular deaths among 8587 patients allocated aspirin *v* 1016 among 8600 allocated placebo; proportional reduction of 23% (SD 4); $P < 0{\cdot}000001$).[1] When these overall results were subdivided by the patients' astrological birth signs, however, no fewer deaths were observed with aspirin than with placebo among patients born under Libra or Gemini (Table 4.2). Although few doctors would consider such analyses to be valid, similarly unreliable conclusions based on "exploratory" data-derived subgroup analyses are widely reported in medical journals and at scientific meetings, and may well have adverse consequences for patient care.

An example of how such subgroup analyses resulted in inappropriate management of patients is provided by the early trials of aspirin for the secondary prevention of stroke. Here, emphasis on the results in men led to a situation where, for almost 20 years, the US Food and Drug Administration approved this use of aspirin only for males; more recent evidence shows this to have been mistaken.[4] A further example is provided by the large Italian GISSI-1 trial comparing streptokinase versus control after acute MI. The overall results favoured streptokinase, but subgroup analyses suggested that streptokinase was beneficial only in patients without prior MI. Fortunately, the GISSI investigators were circumspect about this "finding",[2] and their caution turned out to have been wise, as a subsequent overview of all the large fibrinolytic trials showed that the proportional benefits were similar, irrespective of a history of MI.[21] Many thousands of patients with a previous history of MI might well have been denied fibrinolytic therapy, however, if the apparent pattern of the results in the GISSI-1 subgroups had been believed.

A similar bias may arise in a situation where several studies have addressed much the same therapeutic question but only a few of them are chosen for emphasis. This could be a source of serious bias, as chance fluctuations for or against treatment might affect this choice. It is therefore more appropriate to base inference on a meta-analysis of results from all relevant randomized trials (or, at least, on an unbiased subset of the relevant trials, such as all trials above a certain minimum sample size).[22,23] One additional advantage of such an approach is that such meta-analyses will also minimize random errors, because far more patients (and most importantly, more events) will be available for analysis. The separate trials might well be heterogeneous, but with careful interpretation of such heterogeneity it is often possible to enhance understanding of particular clinical questions.[24] Occasionally, when detailed information on individual patients is available within a really large meta-analysis that includes several thousand major outcomes, such as death[21] or cancer recurrence,[25] it may be feasible to identify particular groups of individuals in whom the benefits or hazards of treatment really are especially great. (Where it has been possible to establish cooperation between trialists before any of the trial results are known, having just a few prespecified subgroup hypotheses can provide some protection against unduly data-dependent emphasis on particular results in a large meta-analysis.[26])

Avoidance of moderate random errors

Small trials may produce false negative results

Whereas the avoidance of moderate biases requires careful attention both to the randomization process and to the analysis and interpretation of the available trial evidence, the avoidance of moderate random errors requires large numbers of events. Because major outcomes such as death may affect only a small proportion of those randomized, very large numbers of patients often need to be studied before the results can be guaranteed to be statistically (and hence medically) convincing. For example, the early trials of intravenous fibrinolytic therapy for acute myocardial infarction were individually too small to provide reliable evidence about any moderate effects of this treatment on mortality, although several did identify an increased risk of serious bleeding. As a result, fibrinolytic therapy was not used routinely until the GISSI-1[2] and ISIS-2[1] "mega-trials" provided such definite evidence of benefit that treatment patterns changed rapidly.[27] It is worth noting, however, that GISSI-1 and ISIS-2 both included more than 10 000 patients and 1000 deaths, but had they only been one tenth as large the observed reduction in mortality would not have been conventionally significant, and would therefore have had much less influence on medical practice.

Table 4.2 Unreliability of "data-dependent" subgroup analyses: ISIS-2 trial of aspirin among over 17 000 patients with suspected acute myocardial infarction[1]

Astrological birth sign	Vascular death by 1 month		*P* value
	Aspirin	Placebo	
Libra or Gemini	150 (11·1%)	147 (10·2%)	0·5
All other signs	654 (9·0%)	869 (12·1%)	<0·0001
Any birth sign	804 (9·4%)	1016 (11·8%)	<0·0001

Small-scale meta-analyses may be unreliable

Because meta-analyses are appearing in medical journals with increasing frequency it is useful to be able to judge the reliability of such reviews – and, in particular, the extent to which confounding, biases or random errors could lead to mistaken conclusions. (In randomized trials, "confounding" exists when a comparison of some particular treatment in one group versus a control group involves the routine coadministration in one group, but not the other, of some cointervention that might affect the outcome.) To avoid any possibility of confounding, and to avoid any flexibility in the question of which trials to consider, meta-analyses should generally include only unconfounded properly randomized trials. The main problems that then remain are those of biases and random errors.

Two types of bias could affect the reliability of a meta-analysis: those that occur within individual trials, and those that relate to the selection of trials. More empirical research into the numerous biases that can occur within randomized trials would be valuable. However, it is clear from existing studies that, for example, inadequate concealment of the likely treatment allocation does quite often result in exaggerated estimates of treatment effect,[28] and that the inappropriate postrandomization exclusion of particular patients is common.[29] Such defects have unpredictable consequences for particular trials, however, and no generalizations about the likely size, or even direction, of the resultant biases are possible.

A further problem involves the process of identifying all relevant trials. Unfortunately, the subset of trials that are eventually published (and hence which are conveniently available) is often a biased sample of the trials that have been done. Trials may well be more likely to be submitted for publication if their results are strikingly positive than if they are negative or null.[30–33] Such "publication bias" can, along with other sources of bias, produce surprisingly impressive looking evidence of effectiveness for treatments that are actually useless.[34] The particular circumstances in which publication bias has contributed to producing misleading estimates of treatment are difficult to identify, and it is still more difficult to generalize about the exact size of any such bias when it does occur.

The problem of incomplete ascertainment is likely to be particularly acute within small meta-analyses that contain no more than a few hundred major outcomes and which consist mainly of small published trials. This is because results from trials with only a limited number of end points are subject to large random errors, and such trials are therefore particularly likely to generate implausibly large effect estimates. If publication bias then results in emphasis on the more promising of these small trial results, the resulting summary odds ratios are likely to be unreliable.[35] Hence, unless the particular circumstances of a small-scale meta-analysis suggest that publication bias is unlikely, it may be best to treat such results as no more than "hypothesis generating". On the other hand, a thoroughly conducted meta-analysis that in aggregate contains sufficient numbers of major outcomes to constitute "large-scale" randomized evidence[4,21,25] is unlikely to be materially affected by publication bias and, provided there are no serious uncontrolled biases (see above) within the individual component trials, is likely to be fairly trustworthy – although, even then, inappropriate subgroup analyses may generate mistaken conclusions.

Large-Scale Randomized Trials

Trials of the effects of treatments on major outcomes can only be made large if they are kept as simple as possible. In particular, as many as possible of the main barriers to rapid recruitment need to be removed. An important way in which trial design can facilitate this is to limit the amount of information that is recorded. For example, data recorded at baseline can often be restricted to important clinical details, including at most only a few major prognostic factors and only a few variables that are thought likely to influence substantially the benefits or hazards of treatment. Similarly, the information recorded at follow up need not be extensive and can be limited largely to those major outcomes that such studies have been designed to assess, and to approximate measures of compliance. (Other outcomes that are of interest but which do not need to be studied on such a large scale may best be assessed in separate smaller studies, or in subsets of these large studies when this is practicable.) Likewise, complicated eligibility criteria, inappropriately detailed consent procedures[36] and unnecessarily extensive auditing of data can all prevent the recruitment of large numbers of patients. Furthermore, if trials are complex they are likely to involve a high cost per patient, which again tends to limit their size. Either way, complexity is rarely a virtue in trials designed to assess major outcomes, whereas simplicity can sometimes lead to the rapid randomization of very large numbers of patients, and to results that change clinical practice within very short periods of time.[1,27]

The "uncertainty principle"

For ethical reasons, randomization is appropriate only if both the doctor and the patient feel substantially uncertain as to which trial treatment is best. The "uncertainty principle" maximizes the potential for recruitment within this ethical constraint (see Box on p 38).

If many hospitals are collaborating in a trial then wholehearted use of the uncertainty principle encourages clinically appropriate heterogeneity in the resulting trial population, and in large trials this may add substantially to the practical value of the results. Among the early trials of

The "uncertainty principle"

A patient can be entered if, and only if, the responsible physician is substantially uncertain as to which of the trial treatments would be most appropriate for that particular patient.

A patient should not be entered if the responsible physician or the patient is, for any medical or non-medical reason, reasonably certain that one of the treatments that might be allocated would be inappropriate for this particular individual (in comparison either with no treatment or with some other treatment that could be offered to the patient in or outside the trial).[37]

fibrinolytic therapy, for example, most of the studies had restrictive entry criteria that precluded the randomization of elderly patients, and so those trials contributed nothing of direct relevance to the important clinical question of whether treatment was useful in older patients. Other trials that did not impose an upper age limit, however, did include some elderly patients, and were therefore able to show that age alone is not a contraindication to fibrinolytic therapy.[21]

Thus, homogeneity of those randomized may be a serious defect in clinical trial design, whereas heterogeneity may be a scientific strength: after all, trials do need to be relevant to a very heterogeneous collection of future patients. The "uncertainty principle" not only ensures ethicality and clinically useful heterogeneity, but also is easily understood and remembered by busy collaborating clinicians, which in turn helps the randomization of large numbers of patients.

Can observational studies substitute for large-scale randomized trials?

As the resources will never be available to design large, simple trials to address all the questions of clinical interest, there have been several recent suggestions that observational studies might be able to provide reliable estimates of the effects of particular treatments. Non-randomized studies do not necessarily provide inaccurate estimates of the effects of treatments, but the point is that they cannot be **guaranteed** to produce reliable estimates because of biases that are inherent in their design. It may well be difficult or impossible to avoid such biases, or to adjust fully for their effects.[38] When non-randomized studies suggest that certain treatments have surprisingly large effects, such findings are often refuted when those treatments are assessed in large randomized trials.[39] For example, the claims of hazards with digoxin in heart failure,[40] based on non-randomized evidence, were not confirmed by the very large randomized DIG (Digitalis Investigation Group) trial.[10] Even if non-randomized comparisons happen to get the right answer then nobody will really know that they have done so. Thus non-randomized studies are of little practical value if the primary aim is to assess moderate treatment effects (whether beneficial or adverse) on major outcomes.

Summary

Many interventions in cardiological practice produce only moderate effects on major outcomes such as death or serious disability. However, even a moderate effect of treatment, if demonstrated clearly enough for that treatment to be widely adopted, can prevent disabling events or death in substantial numbers of people. Moreover, if – as in the treatment of acute myocardial infarction – more than one moderately effective treatment can eventually be identified, then the combination of two or three individually moderate improvements in outcome may collectively result in substantial health gains. In some instances sufficient information is already available from large-scale randomized trials – or, better still, from meta-analyses of those trials – to allow the balance of risk and benefit of particular treatments to be defined for particular patients. But many important questions have still not been answered reliably, and there remains a need for many more large "streamlined" mega-trials, and meta-analyses of such trials, to help resolve some of the outstanding clinical uncertainties in the management of cardiovascular disease.

References

1. ISIS-2 (Second International Study of Infarct Survival) Collaborative Group. Randomised trial of intravenous streptokinase, oral aspirin, both, or neither among 17,187 cases of suspected acute myocardial infarction: ISIS-2. *Lancet* 1988; **ii**:349–60.
2. GISSI (Gruppo Italiano per lo Studio della Streptochinasi nell'infarto miocardico). Effectiveness of intravenous thrombolytic treatment in acute myocardial infarction. *Lancet* 1986;**i**:397–402.
3. Collins R, Peto R, Baigent C, Sleight P. Aspirin, heparin, and fibrinolytic therapy in suspected acute myocardial infarction. *N Engl J Med* 1997;**336**:847–60.
4. Antiplatelet Trialists' Collaboration. Collaborative overview of randomised trials of antiplatelet therapy. I: Prevention of death, myocardial infarction, and stroke by prolonged antiplatelet therapy in various categories of patients. *BMJ* 1994; **308**:81–106.
5. ISIS-4 (Fourth International Study of Infarct Survival) Collaborative Group. ISIS-4: A randomised factorial trial assessing early oral captopril, oral mononitrate, and intravenous magnesium sulphate in 58 050 patients with suspected acute myocardial infarction. *Lancet* 1995;**345**:669–85.
6. Gruppo Italiano per lo Studio della Sopravvivenza nell'Infarto Miocardico. GISSI-3: effects of lisinopril and transdermal glyceryl trinitrate singly and together on 6-week mortality and ventricular function after myocardial infarction. *Lancet* 1994; **343**:1115–22.
7. Chinese Cardiac Study Collaborative Group. Oral captopril versus placebo among 13,634 patients with suspected acute myocardial infarction: interim report from the Chinese Cardiac Study (CCS-1). *Lancet* 1995;**345**:686–7.

8.ISIS-1 (First International Study of Infarct Survival) Collaborative Group. Randomised trial of intravenous atenolol among 16,027 cases of suspected acute myocardial infarction: ISIS-1. *Lancet* 1986;**ii**:57–66.
9.The SOLVD Investigators. Effect of enalapril on survival in patients with reduced left ventricular ejection fractions and congestive heart failure. *N Engl J Med* 1991;**325**:293–302.
10.The Digitalis Investigation Group. The effect of digoxin on mortality and morbidity in patients with heart failure. *N Engl J Med* 1997;**336**:525–33.
11.Collins R, Peto R, Gray R, Parish S. Large-scale randomized evidence: trials and overviews. In: Weatherall D, Ledingham JGG, Warrell DA, eds. *Oxford Textbook of Medicine*, Vol. 1 Oxford: Oxford University Press, 1996.
12.Collins R, MacMahon S. Reliable assessment of the effects of treatment on mortality and major morbidity, I: clinical trials. *Lancet* 2001;**357**:373–80.
13.MacMahon S, Collins R. Reliable assessment of the effects of treatment on mortality and major morbidity, II: observational studies. *Lancet* 2001;**357**:455–62.
14.Armitage P. The role of randomization in clinical trials. *Stat Med* 1982;**1**:345–52.
15.Kunz R, Oxman AD. The unpredictability paradox: review of empirical comparisons of randomised and non-randomised clinical trials. *BMJ* 1998;**317**:1185–90.
16.Hansson L, Lindholm LH, Niskanen L *et al.* for the Captopril Prevention Project (CAPPP) study group. Effect of angiotensin-converting-enzyme inhibition compared with conventional therapy on cardiovascular morbidity and mortality in hypertension: the Captopril Prevention Project (CAPPP) randomised trial. *Lancet* 1999;**353**:611–16.
17.Peto R. Failure of randomisation by "sealed" envelope. *Lancet* 1999;**354**:73.
18.The Coronary Drug Project Research Group. Influence of adherence to treatment and response of cholesterol on mortality in the Coronary Drug Project. *N Engl J Med* 1980;**303**: 1038–41.
19.Peto R, Pike MC, Armitage P *et al.* Design and analysis of randomized clinical trials requiring prolonged observation of each patient. Part I: Introduction and design. *Br J Cancer* 1976;**34**:585–612.
20.Cuzick J, Edwards R, Segnan N. Adjusting for non-compliance and contamination in randomized clinical trials. *Stat Med* 1997;**16**:1017–29.
21.Fibrinolytic Therapy Trialists' Collaborative Group. Indications for fibrinolytic therapy in suspected acute myocardial infarction: collaborative overview of early mortality and major morbidity results from all randomised trials of more than 1000 patients. *Lancet* 1994;**343**:311–22.
22.Collins R, Gray R, Godwin J, Peto R. Avoidance of large biases and large random errors in the assessment of moderate treatment effects: the need for systematic overviews. *Stat Med* 1987;**6**:245–50.
23.Clarke M, Chalmers I. Discussion sections in reports of controlled trials published in general medical journals: islands in search of continents? *JAMA* 1998;**280**:280–2.
24.Thompson SG. Why sources of heterogeneity in meta-analysis should be investigated. *BMJ* 1994;**309**:1351–5.
25.Early Breast Cancer Trialists' Collaborative Group. Systemic treatment of early breast cancer by hormonal, cytotoxic, or immune therapy: 133 randomised trials involving 31 000 recurrences and 24 000 deaths among 75 000 women. *Lancet* 1992;**339**:1–15 (Part I) & 71–85 (Part II).
26.Cholesterol Treatment Trialists' (CTT) Collaboration. Protocol for a prospective collaborative overview of all current and planned randomized trials of cholesterol treatment regimens. *Am J Cardiol* 1995;**75**:1130–4.
27.Collins R, Julian D. British Heart Foundation surveys (1987 and 1989) of United Kingdom treatment policies for acute myocardial infarction. *Br Heart J* 1991;**66**:250–5.
28.Schulz KF, Chalmers I, Hayes RJ, Altman DG. Empirical evidence of bias: dimensions of methodologic quality associated with estimates of treatment effects in controlled trials. *JAMA* 1995;**273**:408–12.
29.Schulz KF, Grimes DA, Altman DG, Hayes RJ. Blinding and exclusions after allocation in randomized controlled trials: survey of published parallel group trials in obstetrics and gynaecology. *BMJ* 1996;**312**:742–4.
30.Dickersin K, Chan S, Chalmers TC *et al.* Publication bias and clinical trials. *Contr Clin Trials* 1987;**8**:343–53.
31.Easterbrook PJ, Berlin JA, Gopelan R, Matthews DR. Publication bias in clinical research. *Lancet* 1991;**337**:867–72.
32.Dickersin K, Min Y-I, Meinert CL. Factors influencing publication of research results. Follow-up of applications submitted to two institutional review boards. *JAMA* 1992;**267**:374–8.
33.Dickersin K, Min Y-I. Publication bias: the problem that won't go away. *Ann NY Acad Sci* 1993;**703**:135–46.
34.Counsell CE, Clarke MJ, Slattery J, Sandercock PAG. The miracle of DICE therapy for acute stroke: fact or fictional product of subgroup analysis. *BMJ* 1994;**309**:1677–81.
35.Davey Smith G, Egger M. Misleading meta-analysis. *BMJ* 1995;**310**:742–54.
36.Doyal L. Journals should not publish research to which patients have not given fully informed consent – with three exceptions. *BMJ* 1997;**314**:1107–11.
37.Collins R, Doll R, Peto R. Ethics of clinical trials. In: Williams CJ, ed. *Introducing New Treatments for Cancer: Practical, Ethical and Legal Problems.* Chichester: John Wiley & Sons, 1992.
38.Sheldon TA. Please bypass the PORT. Observational studies of effectiveness run a poor second to randomised controlled trials. *BMJ* 1994;**309**:142–3.
39.Peto R. Clinical trial methodology. *Biomedicine* Special Issue 1978;**28**:24–36.
40.Yusuf S, Wittes J, Bailey K, Furberg C. Digitalis – a new controversy regarding an old drug: the pitfalls of inappropriate methods. *Circulation* 1986;**73**:13–18.

5 Finding current best evidence to practice evidence-based cardiology

Dereck L Hunt, K Ann McKibbon, R Brian Haynes

Staying current with new diagnostic tests, treatments, and other clinically useful new knowledge in a rapidly evolving field such as cardiology requires effort. Fortunately, this once daunting task is becoming more feasible because of new evidence-based information resources and the steady advance of information technology into clinical settings. This chapter will review ways to find current best evidence for the care of patients with cardiac problems, including both solving patient problems as they arise, and keeping up with new evidence that is ready for application in clinical practice.

The patients whom we see on a daily basis provide an excellent stimulus to staying current. They may have clinical problems that we are unfamiliar with, or that we have not recently reviewed. They may also present us with information from the media or friends to evaluate, or ask us questions that we need to research before answering. Depending on the type of center in which we work, our colleagues, teachers, and students may also ask questions or provide suggestions, making us realize that our knowledge may be "time-challenged".

To become proficient in responding to such challenges (also known as "learning opportunities"), we can make use of a growing array of specialized information resources, aided by information technology that can bring access to our fingertips, almost wherever we may be. To illustrate how patient contacts can provide us with the stimulus to keep up to date and be aware of new evidence, consider the following scenarios.

1. During your outpatient clinic, you see a 56 year old woman who recently became your patient after she moved to your community. She has been diagnosed as having an idiopathic dilated cardiomyopathy and had an echocardiogram 6 months ago that revealed a diffusely enlarged left ventricle with no segmental abnormalities. The ejection fraction was estimated to be less than 30%. You review her current condition and note that her symptoms are controlled on an angiotensin converting enzyme (ACE) inhibitor, digoxin, and a diuretic. Still, she complains of fatigue and dyspnea on moderate exertion. Before leaving, she asks if you can recommend any other medications that would help.
2. Later that day, you pass through the emergency department where an emergency physician happens to notice you. She has been working up a 65 year old man who presented with a swollen left calf. He had an ultrasound that confirmed the presence of a deep venous thrombosis. The patient is anxious to return home because his wife is ill and requires care. The emergency physician is interested in your opinion on the use of low molecular weight heparin for the treatment of deep venous thrombosis in outpatients.

These questions are consistent with the common information needs of physicians. For internists, questions arise at a rate of two questions for every three outpatients seen[1] and five questions on average for every inpatient.[2] No one knows whether cardiologists confront similar numbers of questions, but no professional discipline studied to date is immune from the need to address unanswered questions to keep up with the advance of knowledge.

How would you address each of the questions raised by the clinical scenarios? The possibilities include using an electronic bibliographic database such as MEDLINE, a specialized abstract journal like *ACP Journal Club* or *Evidence-Based Cardiovascular Medicine*, a current textbook, or the Cochrane Library. We will consider the strengths and weaknesses of these resources and apply them to the clinical problems.

MEDLINE

MEDLINE is a huge, multipurpose database of medical literature citations and abstracts produced by the US National Library of Medicine (NLM). It includes citations to almost all important clinical studies, and also a much larger volume of non-clinical studies and articles. Few other resources currently rival this scope. Accessing MEDLINE is relatively easy.[3–5] CD Rom based systems, online systems, and, most importantly, internet access are all available. Examples of CD Rom systems include OVID, Aries, SilverPlatter, and DIALOG. Online access by modem is available through vendors such as PaperChase and HealthGate.[6] Internet access is readily available (see Medical Matrix (http://www. medmatrix.org) and Dr Felix's Free MEDLINE Page (http://www.beaker.iupui. edu/drfelix) sites for locations that offer MEDLINE access). Some of these MEDLINE systems have user fees but, at least at present, free access is available from many, led by the NLM PubMed (http://www.ncbi.nlm.nih.gov/PubMed/) internet site. This site features the earliest MEDLINE access to newly published articles and point-and-click search strategies that improve the yield of clinically useful studies on the cause, course, diagnosis, and treatment of clinical problems.

If ready access is one of MEDLINE's strengths, the skills needed to rapidly and dependably locate high quality articles that specifically address a clinical question are a weakness. A working knowledge of MEDLINE searching terminology and searching strategies is essential. Luckily, most hospital and university libraries offer training courses for MEDLINE. The NLM has also established a set of eight regional medical libraries that are charged with providing access and training for all US health personnel (+1-800-338-7657). Physicians in the UK can call the Health Care Information Service (+44-207-412-7477) for similar information, while Canadians can call the Canada Institute for Scientific and Technical Information (+1-800-668-1222).

Turning to our initial scenario, we are interested in locating information about new medical therapies for patients with idiopathic dilated cardiomyopathy. Also, it would be wise to focus initially on treatments that already have been adequately tested in well-designed clinical trials.[7] While it may be interesting to read about new medications that are being designed and tested at the laboratory level, or are undergoing early human testing, this information will not be immediately applicable in our clinical practices.

Turning to MEDLINE for assistance, we might begin searching by using a medical subject heading (MeSH) for congestive heart failure. MEDLINE indexers choose appropriate terms from a thesaurus of 14 000 specific terms and 18 000 synonyms for content and methodology. Unfortunately, these terms are not always intuitive (for example, β blockers indexed as adrenergic β antagonists). Therefore, it is often necessary to search through the MeSH vocabulary before carrying out a search. The software for all search systems includes MeSH, so it is quite easy to search for appropriate terms. For our topic, a search for CONGESTIVE HEART FAILURE leads to HEART FAILURE, CONGESTIVE.

Depending on the topic and the scope that you are interested in covering, you may also want to take advantage of two additional features of MeSH headings. Because many articles deal predominantly with two or three topics, the NLM will indicate these topics for each citation by designating them as major subjects of the article. Limiting your search to articles in which the search term has been designated as the major subject heading will be beneficial if you retrieve too many citations from using the search term without "majoring" it. Sometimes, though, you can miss important studies this way. A trial and error approach may be needed to retrieve the best studies.

"Exploding" is another useful feature of MEDLINE MeSH indexing. When articles are indexed, they are classified according to the most specific MeSH heading available. Thus, if you wish to identify all articles that deal with congestive heart failure, including those with more specific MeSH terms such as congestive cardiomyopathy, then you can do so by searching with the term EXPLODE HEART FAILURE, CONGESTIVE.

If you are searching for a topic that has not been well indexed, you may want to take advantage of textword searching. Using this approach, you are simply asking MEDLINE to search the titles and abstracts of all the citations for any occurrences of a certain sequence of letters, such as "dilated". This approach is particularly useful for new drugs or concepts that have not yet been incorporated into MeSH. MeSH is updated annually, but the lag can be considerably longer for certain terms.

If several different endings to a word may have been used, and you wish to identify them all, you can use "truncation", using the "*" symbol. For example, if you asked for RANDOM*, MEDLINE would search for RANDOM, RANDOMIZATION, RANDOMIZED, RANDOMISATION, RANDOMISED, and RANDOMLY. Be careful with truncation. The term "salmon*" retrieves not only the fish but salmonella as well! Some systems may use symbols other than "*", such as ":" or "?".

Returning to identifying new therapies for patients with significant left ventricular dysfunction, EXPLODE HEART FAILURE, CONGESTIVE is a good start, but we need to narrow in on treatments that have been tested in well-designed studies. Luckily, a number of methodological search strategies have been tested and validated for retrieving sound studies for questions relating to therapy, prognosis, etiology or cause, and diagnosis (Box 5.1).[8,9] Alternatively, you can search for a systematic review of studies. Research is currently ongoing to establish the best approach to identify systematic reviews and meta-analyses.[10] For our current search, limiting the citations to systematic reviews and meta-analyses seemed like a reasonable first step. A simple but not fully validated strategy to identify systematic reviews and meta-analyses is to identify all citations in which the publication type is designated as meta-analysis (note that in addition to indexing articles according to subject, the NLM also indexes citations according to "publication type"). Over 40 publication types are recognized, including "meta-analysis", "randomized controlled trial", and "review"), as well as citations that include the phrase "meta-anal*" as a textword, and citations that are designated as reviews in the publication type section, but also have the textword "MEDLINE" in their abstract. Putting this all together yielded the search strategy in Box 5.2 using PubMed.

Box 5.1 Optimal search strategies for identifying studies relating to treatment, diagnosis, prognosis, or etiology using MEDLINE

- **Treatment**
  - *Best single term:* clinical trial.pt. ("pt" indicates publication type)
    Combination of terms with best specificity: placebo:.tw. ("tw" indicates textword) OR double.tw. AND blind:.tw.
    Combination of terms with best sensitivity: randomized controlled trial.pt. OR random:.tw. OR drug therapy (as a subheading of the subject) OR therapeutic use (as a subheading of the subject)
- **Diagnosis**
  - *Best single term:* explode diagnosis
    Combination of terms with best specificity: explode "sensitivity and specificity" OR predictive.tw. AND value:.tw.
    Combination of terms with best sensitivity: explode "sensitivity and specificity" OR explode diagnosis (as a subheading of the subject) OR sensitivity.tw. OR specificity.tw. OR diagnostic use (as a subheading of the subject)
- **Prognosis**
  - *Best single term:* explode cohort studies
    Combination of terms with best specificity: prognosis OR survival analysis
    Combination of terms with best sensitivity: incidence OR explode mortality OR follow up studies OR prognos:.tw. OR predict:.tw. OR course:.tw. OR mortality (as a subheading of the subject)
- **Etiology or cause**
  - *Best single term:* risk.tw.
    Combination of terms with best specificity: cohort studies OR case–control studies
    Combination of terms with best sensitivity: explode cohort studies OR explode risk OR odds.tw. AND ratio:.tw. OR relative.tw. AND risk:.tw. OR case.tw. AND control:.tw.

Based on Haynes *et al*[8] and Wilczynski *et al*[9]

Box 5.2

1.	Heart failure, congestive	41 251	(PubMed automatically explodes MeSH terms)
2.	Meta-analysis[pt]	6123	(pt indicates publication type)
3.	Meta-anal*[tw]	9683	(tw indicates textword)
4.	Review[pt] AND medline[tw]	5156	
5.	#2 OR #3 OR #4	16 637	(the "OR" means that all citations in either #2 or #3 or #4 will be included)
6.	#1 AND #5	141	(the "AND" means that only citations that occur in both #1 and #5 will be identified)

Looking at the titles and abstracts of these articles, you find that one is a meta-analysis on β blockers, and the abstract suggests that these medications are almost certainly beneficial. You decide to go to the library to retrieve this paper,[11] and then to critically appraise it using the guidelines for a systematic review.[12]

Many alternative ways exist for conducting a MEDLINE search, including the one just displayed. Unfortunately, because no perfect recipe exists, what works well in one situation may not work as well in another. Combining an appropriate content term (HEART FAILURE, CONGESTIVE, in this case) with methods terms for reviews (as above) or for sound study designs (as in Box 5.1) is a good place to start. It also has to be considered, however, that such searches are bound to take some time. This is because of the general nature of this huge biomedical research database: it is so large and comprehensive that even the extensive indexing and care that is taken in preparing it are insufficient to guarantee quick and accurate retrieval for clinical uses. Fortunately, many vendors have developed specialized subsets of MEDLINE for clinical use in cardiology. For example, Aries (http://www.kfinder.com) offers a cardiovascular disease subset (CardLine) on compact disc that you can subscribe to yourself. Instead of having 1 full year of MEDLINE on each CD Rom disc, these subsets provide journals and citations relating to a specific field for inclusion. For example, CardLine has cardiology citations from MEDLINE for the 10 most recent years on one disc.

Specialized clinical information resources

While large electronic bibliographic databases such as MEDLINE can be very helpful, they can also be very frustrating or overwhelming because of the different ways that articles can be indexed and because of the vast array of preclinical and non-clinical literature that is included. MEDLINE serves many user groups besides clinicians (basic scientists and other researchers, educators, librarians, journalists, etc.). An alternative is to use a resource that includes only methodologically sound and clinically relevant articles, such as *ACP Journal Club* (American College of Physicians (ACP-ASIM)), for internal medicine and its subspecialties, *Evidence-Based Medicine* (for all major specialties; from ACP-ASIM and from the BMJ Publishing Group), and the cardiology journal *Evidence-Based Cardiovascular Medicine* (published by Churchill Livingstone). These are available in both paper and electronic versions. In addition to including only methodologically sound articles[13] and presenting the results using a structured abstract format, these journals also include a commentary written by a clinical expert, designed to put the study findings into clinical context.

Searching *ACP Journal Club* (www.acpjc.org) using the text phrase "low molecular weight heparin" locates several relevant references, including one directly on target.[14] This report summarizes the findings of two randomized controlled trials comparing intravenous heparin administered in hospital with subcutaneous low molecular weight heparin administered at home, and both found that outpatient therapy was as safe and effective as inhospital management.

Other resources

The Cochrane Library is an increasingly valuable source of evidence summaries and trials of healthcare interventions. This new electronic database is updated quarterly and contains the collected work of the Cochrane Collaboration, an international voluntary organization that prepares, maintains, and disseminates systematic reviews of randomized trials of healthcare interventions. Available on CD Rom and via the internet (http://www.cochranelibrary.com), the Cochrane Library consists of three key sections for locating clinical evidence: the Cochrane Database of Systematic Reviews (CDSR), the Database of Abstracts of Reviews of Effectiveness (DARE), and the Cochrane Controlled Trials Registry (CCTR). The CDSR consists of the full reports of Cochrane Collaboration systematic reviews as well as protocols for ongoing systematic reviews. DARE is produced by the UK National Health Services Center for Reviews and Dissemination located at the University of York. It contains citations to many non-Cochrane systematic reviews, and includes structured abstracts for many of them. The CCTR is a growing collection of over 320 000 citations to therapeutic intervention trials.

Searching the Cochrane Library is relatively easy and requires only entering a word or short phrase. The Library automatically searches all three sections for any relevant reviews or citations. Applying this to our scenarios, searching using the term "dilated cardiomyopathy" in Cochrane Library 2001, Issue 4, yields numerous citations: three citations to completed reviews in the CDSR, seven citations in the DARE, and 267 citations in the CCTR. The Cochrane reviews address the role of anticoagulation, antiplatelet agents, and digoxin in patients with a cardiomyopathy, and the structured abstracts within the DARE include a meta-analysis of β blocker studies.[15] Doing a similar search using the term "low molecular weight heparin" locates numerous references including a Cochrane review entitled "Home versus in-patient treatment for deep vein thrombosis".[16] This systematic review was updated in February 2001 and identified the two studies that were found earlier using *ACP Journal Club*.

Textbooks

At this point, you may be thinking about your textbooks. What role do these have in clinical practice and in particular with respect to staying current? Textbooks remain an important resource for clinicians in terms of anatomy and pathophysiology, the basics of practice that usually do not change very quickly, except perhaps for molecular biology. They also provide descriptions of the classic presentations of numerous disease conditions and review important aspects of the history, physical examination, and diagnostic testing. By reviewing conditions that may present with similar findings, a good textbook can also help to broaden the differential diagnosis in more complex cases. These references may also describe medication adverse effects and pharmacokinetics, and may include historical perspectives and practical suggestions to assist in patient management.

Textbooks, however, are seldom explicit about the quality or currency of evidence used in recommendations for management. Also, there is often a passage of 3 or more years between updates of specialty textbooks, and new studies may have been published in the interval. Particularly for rapidly evolving aspects of management such as laboratory diagnosis and therapeutics, print textbooks simply cannot be trusted. Fortunately, we are now seeing the emergence of CD Rom and Internet versions of textbooks with regular updates, such as UpToDate[17] and *Scientific American Medicine* (SAM).[18]

The internet

This brings us to the world wide web, an increasingly useful resource for locating current information, and one that our patients are accessing at an increasing rate. We have already mentioned how MEDLINE, *ACP Journal Club* and the Cochrane Library can be accessed over the web. A rapidly growing number of journals are also available online. A few examples include the *New England Journal of Medicine* (http://www.nejm.org), *Annals of Internal Medicine* (http://www.acponline.org), *JAMA* (http://jama.ama-assn.org), *BMJ* (http://www.bmj.com), and *The Lancet* (www. thelancet. com). A number of cardiology textbooks are also available over the internet, as are many clinical practice guidelines. Two websites that have extensive cardiology sections are the Medscape (http://www.medscape.com) and Medical Matrix (http://www.medmatrix.org) sites.

Journals and browsing to keep up to date

We have focused to this point on looking for evidence when it is needed. If the search is successful, the evidence can be applied immediately and this can be a powerful learning experience. But what if we don't search for evidence because we don't know that we are out of date? A complementary strategy is needed, browsing the medical literature regularly in one way or another. The difficulty is that so many journals include articles relevant to cardiology that it is impracticable to review them all. One of the best solutions is to subscribe to a journal such as *Evidence-Based Cardiovascular Medicine* that continuously scans a wide range of journals in a systematic way, according to explicit criteria, and includes structured abstracts and commentaries on methodologically sound and clinically relevant studies.

Conclusion

In summary, while the time that we devote to updating ourselves with new developments is limited, a growing number of easy-access resources are available so that we can use this time effectively. MEDLINE is more readily available now than ever, and is seeding the development of specialty-specific collections. Journals that abstract only high-quality, clinically relevant articles are appearing, and systematic reviews are becoming the norm. Internet-accessible textbooks that are regularly updated are also becoming available. Applying these resources to clinical care on an ongoing basis after appraising the quality of information and considering how it relates to our individual patient's circumstances can lead to improvements in the quality of care we provide.

Key points

- New resources are rapidly emerging that make keeping up to date with clinically significant developments in cardiology easier than ever.
- Large bibliographic databases, such as MEDLINE, are becoming more accessible to practicing physicians, and search strategies for locating high quality studies are now available.
- Specialty journals, such as *Evidence-Based Cardiovascular Medicine*, that identify and abstract methodologically sound and clinically relevant studies, also facilitate the ongoing process of staying current.

References

1. Covell DG, Uman GC, Manning PR. Information needs in office practice: are they being met? *Ann Intern Med* 1985; **103**:596–9.
2. Osherof JA, Forsythe DE, Buchanan BG *et al.* Physicians' information needs: analysis of questions posed during clinical teaching. *Ann Intern Med* 1991;**114**:576–81.
3. McKibbon KA, Walker-Dilks CJ, Beyond *ACP Journal Club*: how to harness MEDLINE to solve clinical problems (Editorial). *ACP J Club* 1994;**120**:A10–12.
4. Haynes RB, Walker CJ, McKibbon KA, Johnston M, Willan A. Performance of 27 MEDLINE systems tested by searches on clinical questions. *J Am Med Informatics Assoc* 1994;**1**: 285–95.
5. Engstrom P. MEDLINE free-for-all spurs questions about search value: who pays? *Medicine on the NET* 1996;**2**:1–5.
6. Haynes RB, McKibbon KA, Walker CJ *et al.* Online access to MEDLINE in clinical settings. A study of use and usefulness. *Ann Intern Med* 1990;**112**:78–84.
7. Sackett DL, Richardson SR, Rosenberg W, Haynes RB. *Evidence-based medicine: how to practise and teach EBM.* London: Churchill Livingstone, 1997.
8. Haynes RB, Wilczynski N, McKibbon KA, Walker CJ, Sinclair JC. Developing optimal search strategies for detecting clinically sound studies in MEDLINE. *J Am Med Informatics Assoc* 1994;**1**:447–58.
9. Wilczynski NL, MWalker CJ, McKibbon KA, Haynes RB. Assessment of methodological search filters in MEDLINE. *Proc Ann Symp Comp Appl Med Care* 1994;**17**:601–5.

10.Hunt DL, McKibbon KA. Locating and appraising systematic reviews. *Ann Intern Med* 1997;**126**:532–8.
11.Brophy JM, Joseph L, Rouleau JL. β-blockers in congestive heart failure. A bayesian meta-analysis. *Ann Intern Med* 2001;**134**:550–60.
12.Oxman A, Cook D, Guyatt G. Users' guides to the medical literature. VI. How to use an overview. *JAMA* 1994;**272**:1367–71.
13.Haynes RB. The origins and aspirations of *ACP Journal Club* (Editorial). *ACP J Club* 1991;**114**:A18.
14.Low-molecular-weight heparin at home was as effective as unfractionated heparin in the hospital in proximal DVT (Abstracts). *ACP J Club* 1996;**125**:2–3. [Abstracts of Koopman MM, Prandoni P, Piovella F *et al.* Treatment of venous thrombosis with intravenous unfractionated heparin administered in the hospital as compared with subcutaneous low-molecular-weight heparin administered at home. *N Engl J Med* 1996; **334**:682–7; and Levine M, Gent M, Hirsh J *et al.* A comparison of low-molecular-weight heparin administered primarily at home with unfractionated heparin administered in the hospital for proximal deep-vein thrombosis. *N Engl J Med* 1996;**334**:677–81.]
15.Zarembsk DG, Nolan PE Jr, Slack MK, Lui CY. Meta-analysis of the use of low-dose beta-adrenergic blocking therapy in idiopathic or ischemic dilated cardiomyopathy. *Am J Cardiol* 1996;**77**:1247–50.
16.Schraibman IG, Milne AA, Royle EM. Home versus in-patient treatment for deep vein thrombosis (Cochrane Review). In: *The Cochrane Library*, Issue 4, 2001. Oxford: Update Software.
17.Rose BD, ed. *UpToDate*. Wellesley, MA: UpToDate, Inc., 2001.
18.Dale DC, Federman DD, eds. *Scientific American Medicine*. New York: Scientific American Medicine, 1978–97.

6 Understanding concepts related to health economics

Mark Hlatky

Introduction

Economics is concerned with how to allocate scarce resources among alternative uses efficiently and effectively. It is a fundamental principle of economics that resources are limited relative to human wants, and that those resources have alternative uses.[1] Consequently, when people say that the cost of health care has grown too high, they mean that the quantity of resources flowing toward medical care has grown to the point where additional funds cannot be spent on other things that society values, such as education, public safety, environmental protection, public works, pensions for the retired or disabled, or assistance to the poor. The fact that most people put a very high value on health does not mean that they are willing to provide limitless resources to medical care. Indeed, even the goal of improving health and longevity may also be served by non-medical expenditures on programs such as nutritional supplements, a safe and clean water supply, police and fire protection, or safety improvements to roads, as well as by medical expenditures.

The cost of medical care has been rising steadily for the past 50 years, but it has only been in the past decade that the level of expenditures became so large as to cause alarm among policy makers, payers, and the general public (Table 6.1). The steady expansion of health care has now begun to meet substantial resistance in the large industrial countries, and new policies and payment mechanisms have been introduced to contain the rising cost of medical care. As a consequence, physicians must now consider cost as they design programs to prevent, diagnose, and treat disease. Cardiovascular diseases consume a large share of health care resources (Table 6.2), so cardiovascular specialists must be particularly knowledgeable about health economics. This chapter will attempt to outline the major principles of health economics relevant to cardiovascular medicine. First, some general concepts of health economics will be presented. Second, methods to identify and compare the costs of cardiovascular interventions will be described. Finally, the principles of cost effectiveness analysis will be discussed.

Table 6.1 US national healthcare expenditures, 2000

Category	US$ (×10⁹)	Percentage
Hospital care	412·1	32
Physician services	286·4	22
Other professional services	99·0	8
Drugs, supplies	171·5	13
Nursing home care	92·2	7
Home health care	32·4	2
Other personal health care	36·7	3
Administration	80·9	6
Public health	44·2	3
Research	25·3	2
Construction	18·6	1
Total	1299·5	100

Source: *Health Affairs* 2002;**21**:207–18

Table 6.2 Resources devoted to cardiovascular care in the USA

Category	n (×10³)	Percentage (of total)
Deaths[a]	934	39
Hospital admissions[b]	6344	20
Myocardial infarction	829	
Heart failure	962	
Cerebrovascular disease	961	
Operations and procedures[b]	6133	15
Cardiac catheterization	1271	
Coronary bypass surgery	355	
Coronary angioplasty	599	
Pacemaker-related	336	
Physician office visits[c]	59 996	8
Electrocardiograms	22 596	
Prescriptions[c]	176 839	16

Sources: [a] NCHS Monthly Vital Statistics Report 2001; **49**:12
[b] NCHS Advance Data 2001 (No. 319)
[c] NCHS Advance Data 2001 (No. 322)

General concepts

Various societies have adopted different systems to pay for health care, and these systems reflect societal values and the historical experience within each country. The United Kingdom has a national health service, Canada has national health insurance, France and Germany have public/private financing for health care, and the United States has a perplexing and rapidly evolving patchwork of public and private health insurance systems. These are very different systems to finance health care, and yet each is faced with the same issues of how to allocate the limited resources available to best provide health care. Each country is also facing the same steady rise of healthcare costs, despite the wide differences in the ways they finance health care.

Provision of cardiovascular services requires resources in all societies, irrespective of the method of financing or delivering health care. Coronary bypass surgery, for example, is very resource-intensive, with the operation requiring cardiac surgeons, a cardiac anesthesiologist or anesthetist, a perfusionist, several nurses, and considerable quantities of specialized supplies and equipment. Postoperative care also requires skilled nurses and physicians, with support from specialized supplies, equipment, and facilities. Each health professional involved in cardiac surgery spends the scarce resource of time to care for the patient – time that could be put to other valuable uses, such as care for other patients. The drugs used, the disposable supplies, the operating room equipment, even the hospital building, all cost money. All of these are true costs to the system, even if the coronary bypass operation is performed "for free" – that is, without charge to the patient. The scene in the operating room, the postoperative recovery areas, and the hospital wards is much the same in the United Kingdom, Canada, France, Germany, and the United States despite the different ways these societies pay for medical care. The resources used in the care of patients, and the increasing sophistication of that care, drive healthcare costs up in each of these countries, irrespective of the way such care is paid for.

Another basic concept of economics is the so-called "law of diminishing returns". This concept is illustrated in Figure 6.1, in which the quantity of resources used in health care is plotted on the horizontal axis, and the resulting health benefits on the vertical axis. In the case of the patient with an acute myocardial infarction, for example, survival would be improved as more resources are applied, such as prehospital transportation, electrocardiographic monitoring, access to defibrillation, and a competent team to deliver coronary care. Outcomes might be further improved by reperfusion therapy, but with a greater increment in survival from using a cheaper, basic approach (streptokinase, for example) relative to no therapy, than from more expensive alternatives (such as tissue plasminogen activator (tPA) or PTCA). The extra benefit from adding even more aggressive care will be smaller still, and at some point the patient may be harmed by overly aggressive care. Helping physicians define the optimal point on this curve (Figure 6.1) is one of the goals of economic analysis.

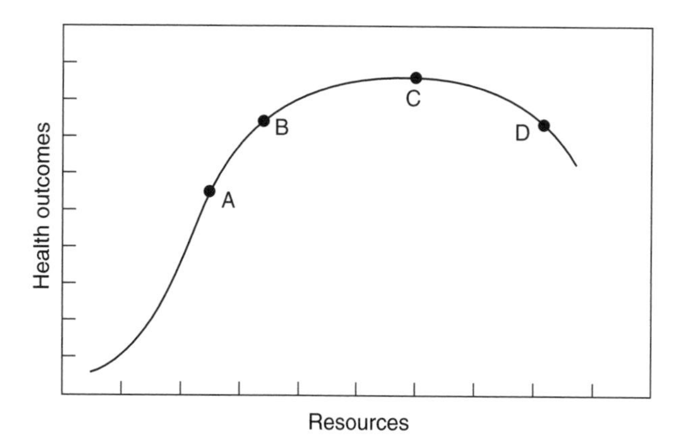

Figure 6.1 General relationship between increasing healthcare resources (horizontal axis) and health outcomes (vertical axis). At point A, outcomes are improving rapidly with increased resources and treatment is cost effective. At point B, outcomes are still improving with increased resources, but at a rate that is not cost effective. At point C, increased resources are no longer improving outcome (that is, "flat of the curve"), and at point D increased resources actually lead to worse outcomes, through iatrogenic complications and overtreatment.

Determination of costs

The cost of producing a particular healthcare service can be defined in a variety of ways. The cost of performing a coronary angiogram can be used as a specific example that will illustrate the various aspects of cost and how the cost might be measured. Performing a coronary angiogram requires a variety of resources, including radiographic equipment, trained personnel (including an angiographer and technical assistants), and specialized supplies such as catheters, radiographic contrast, and sterile drapes. The equipment needed is very expensive to purchase, and the healthcare facility where it is installed may require special renovations to assure proper radiation shielding and adequate electrical power. The capital cost for a coronary angiography laboratory will be considerable, perhaps $2–3 million, depending on the type of equipment purchased. The laboratory will have a physical lifespan of perhaps 7–10 years, although technologic innovations may lead to replacement of the equipment before the end of its physical lifespan. The cost of building an angiography suite represents a large *fixed cost* for coronary angiography, a cost that is roughly the same whether the laboratory performs 200 or 2000 angiograms per year. The cost per case is lower in the high volume laboratory, however, because the fixed equipment costs can be spread over more cases. Thus, if the equipment costs

$2·5 million and has a useful life of 10 years, the prorated share of fixed costs for each patient in the low volume laboratory performing 200 cases per year is

$$\text{Fixed costs/case} = \frac{\$2\,500\,000}{(200 \text{ cases/yr})(10 \text{ years})} = \$1250/\text{case}$$

whereas in the high volume laboratory (2000 cases per year) the prorated share of fixed costs per case would be

$$\text{Fixed costs/case} = \frac{\$2\,500\,000}{(2000 \text{ cases/yr})(10 \text{ years})} = \$125/\text{case}$$

Procedures that have high fixed costs will be performed with greater economic efficiency in centers that have sufficient volume to spread those fixed costs over a larger number of individual patients. (There may be additional advantages to larger procedure volumes as well, since the technical proficiency is higher and clinical outcomes of many procedures are usually better when performed in higher volume clinical centers.)[2–4] Procedures with lower fixed costs will have a smaller effect of volume on costs.

In contrast to the fixed equipment costs, the cost of supplies consumed in performing coronary angiography varies directly with the volume of cases performed, and the supply cost per case will be fairly constant irrespective of the volume of cases performed (apart from the small effect of discounts available to large volume purchasers). The cost of laboratory staff falls in between these two extremes, in that the hours worked in the catheterization laboratory by technical staff can be varied somewhat according to the volume of cases performed, but some staff effort is required regardless of patient volumes, such as supervisors.

Hospital overhead is also a real cost, but one that is less directly linked to any one medical service or procedure. Hospitals must pay for admitting offices, the medical records department, central administration, the laundry service, the cafeteria, housekeeping and utilities, to name just a few areas. These costs cannot be tied easily to the coronary angiography procedure in the same way as the cost of the catheters or radiographic contrast. Most facilities assign a share of these costs to patient care services according to a formula such as the step down method. Discussion of specific methods to allocate hospital overhead is beyond the scope of this chapter, but can be found in several articles and books.[5,6]

The overall effect of procedure volume on the cost per case is illustrated in Figure 6.2. In general, the cost per case declines as more cases are performed, up to the limit of the facility's capacity (for example, 2000 cases). If volume increases further, more facilities must be built, increasing the cost per case, as more fixed costs are spread over a few more patients. Figure 6.2 also illustrates the distinction between concepts of "marginal cost" and long run "average cost". The marginal cost is the added cost of doing one more case. In an already equipped and staffed coronary angiography laboratory, the marginal cost of performing one more

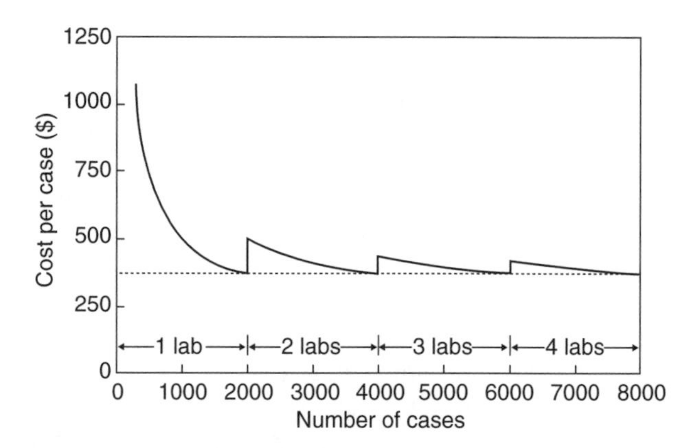

Figure 6.2 Cost per case for coronary angiography as a function of clinical volume. Assumes fixed costs per laboratory of $250 000 per year, and marginal (that is, variable) costs of $250 per case. When volume reaches 2000 cases per year in a laboratory, the model assumes an additional laboratory will be built. The dotted line indicates the "long run average" cost per case of $375.

procedure is just the cost of the disposable supplies consumed in the case: the catheters, radiographic contrast, and other sterile supplies. In the example of Figure 6.2, the marginal cost is $250 per case. The marginal cost is lower than the average cost per case ($375 per case), which also includes a prorated share of the salaries of the laboratory staff, depreciation of the laboratory equipment costs, and the facility's overhead costs.

Costs *v* charges

Costs and charges are related but distinct concepts. The cost of a medical service represents the value of the resources required to produce it. The charge for a service is a specific form of reimbursement to healthcare providers in a fee-for-service healthcare system. The cost and charge for providing a service should be quite close to one another in a competitive economic market. The reason is simple: if one provider charged an amount much higher than it actually cost to provide a service, a competitor could offer the same service at a lower price and still come out ahead. Conversely, if a provider charged less than the costs of production, the provider would lose money. These basic economic principles have not applied very well to medical care, at least until recently, because medical care has not had significant competition on prices.

In regulated or non-price competitive healthcare systems, the charge (price) for a service need not bear a close relationship to the cost of producing a service. Hospitals might choose to set high prices for some services, such as coronary bypass surgery, and use the excess revenues to subsidize other services that were less well reimbursed, such as the emergency department or, in academic centers, medical education, and research. With greater price sensitivity on the part of healthcare payers, the subsidization of one medical service with the proceeds of another service has been sharply curtailed. While this trend has had the positive effect of bringing an element of economic reality to medicine, it has also caused dislocations and considerable harm as worthwhile endeavors have lost the funding they previously enjoyed from cross-subsidization. In the long run, medical education, clinical research, and services to uninsured or poorly insured patients should receive direct funding to replace the indirect funding by cross-subsidies, but in the transition these endeavors have been threatened due to loss of a traditional funding base.

Estimation of costs

The cost of providing a specific service, such as coronary bypass surgery, can be established in several alternative ways. In principle, one valid way to measure cost would be to identify a competitive market for medical service, and note the charge (price) for coronary bypass surgery in that market. While competitive market pricing might work well for commodities such as consumer electronic devices or farm products, it is not well suited to medical care, where there are few competitive markets. An alternative method to measure cost is to take note of the charge for a service, and apply correction factors to estimate cost more accurately. A third method to estimate costs is to examine in detail the resources used to provide a service, and apply price weights to the resources used:

$$\text{Cost}_j = \sum_i (\text{Quantity})_{ij} \times (\text{Price})_{ij}$$

The use of these different approaches to cost determination is illustrated by a study that estimated the costs savings achievable by substituting coronary angioplasty for coronary bypass surgery.[7] In that study, hospital billing records were used to construct resource consumption profiles for patients undergoing either angioplasty or bypass surgery for the treatment of stable angina. A microcosting approach was then applied to the resource consumption profiles, with the cost of a specific resource (for example, an electrocardiogram) defined either as the cost of supplies only (marginal cost or variable cost) or as the cost of supplies, personnel and equipment, but omitting overhead (average direct cost). Charges on the billing record for a service were also converted to costs by two different correction factors, also known as ratios of cost to charges. One cost–charge ratio included all direct costs of providing a service (supplies, personnel, and equipment), but omitted hospital overhead (for example, medical records, laundry, utilities, administration). The second cost–charge ratio allocated a share of hospital overhead to each service in addition to its direct costs.

As shown in Table 6.3, the cost savings attributable to substitution of angioplasty for bypass surgery varied considerably according to how costs were defined. The lowest cost savings are evident when only marginal costs are included, and fixed cost and overhead excluded. The average direct cost difference is intermediate in value, and comparable estimates of this cost savings were obtained from the use of resource consumption profiles and cost weights (method 2) or the cost-to-charge ratio method that omitted overhead (method 3). Finally, the inclusion of overhead (method 4) led to the highest absolute difference in costs.

The differences in cost as estimated using these methods is directly related to the issue of how the information is to be used or, put another way, depends on the answer to the question, "cost to whom?". A hospital manager might be most interested in the marginal cost of procedures (method 1) in looking at the effect of adding or subtracting a small number of cases to the volume performed in an institution. Under a fixed budget for cardiac services, for instance, the effect of substituting angioplasty for bypass surgery may be small, given that the personnel, equipment, and overhead are largely fixed. Performing a few extra procedures with existing facilities adds very little cost from the perspective of the

Table 6.3 Effect of different definitions of cost on the savings possible by substitution of coronary angioplasty for bypass surgery

Definition of cost	PTCA cost ($)	CABG cost ($)	Difference ($)	PTCA/CABG ratio (%)
Variable cost only	2672	4607	1935	58
Average direct cost				
By microcosting	4073	8666	4593	47
By ratio of cost-to-charges	4935	10281	5346	48
Average cost + overhead	7530	15367	7837	49
Charges	9556	19644	10088	49

Source: adapted from Hlatky *et al*[7]

head of a clinical service or a hospital manager. They may even be willing to perform a modest number of additional cases at a reimbursement level below their actual average cost, but above marginal cost, in order to increase volume and spread their fixed costs over more patients. Thus, marginal or variable costs are quite relevant to decision makers within the institution providing a service.

The perspective of a policy maker or health planner includes a longer time horizon and the possibility of adding or subtracting substantial volumes of clinical services. From this perspective, no cost is truly fixed, for personnel needs can be adjusted, and the number of facilities providing a service can be altered. This perspective is a broader one, and the costs considered are therefore more inclusive. For most policy level discussions, long run average cost is the most relevant measure.

International perspectives

With the advent of large multicenter clinical trials that enroll patients from several countries, interest has developed in cost comparisons between countries for the same service. Cost estimation as part of large randomized trials will enhance clinical decision making, for the randomized design is the strongest way to compare all outcomes of therapeutic alternatives, including cost. Extension of cost comparisons across national borders introduces a number of technical and conceptual issues that deserve discussion.

Different countries measure cost in their respective national currencies, so that readers in another country need to convert between units (for example, pounds sterling or euros to US dollars). These conversions can be done using currency exchange rates, or the closely related purchasing power parity factors. The differences between countries in units of measurement are important, but this issue is fairly simple to address.

A more thorny issue in international comparisons is differences in the relative prices of the resources used to provide a service and differences in resource profiles used to provide a service. Thus, if the cost of service *j* is defined as

$$\text{Cost}_j = \sum_i (\text{Quantity})_{ij} \times (\text{Price})_{ij}$$

then cost may differ among countries due to either differences in the quantity of resources used to provide a service, price differentials for the same resources, or both. A specific example will help illustrate these concepts (Table 6.4). Care of a patient with acute myocardial infarction given thrombolysis includes the cost of the drug, the cost of basic hospital care, and the cost of additional tests and treatments in the convalescent phase. Table 6.4 presents hypothetical costs of basic care in two countries, with monetary values expressed in dollar units for simplicity. The costs of drugs in Country 1 are higher than in Country 2, where drug prices are strictly regulated. The time spent by the hospital staff to care for the patient are quite similar in Country 1 and Country 2 (50 hours per patient for Treatment A and 54 for Treatment B, a difference due to lower complication rates with Treatment A). The average hourly compensation for hospital staff is, however, higher in Country 2, so that total personnel costs are higher as well. Thus, both cost savings and the relative costs of Treatment A and B are different in these two healthcare systems, due to different prices for the same resources used to care for a myocardial infarct patient.

There may also be differences in the level of resource use between countries, especially for discretionary procedures such as coronary angiography. Suppose that the use of Treatment A cuts the use of coronary angiography by one third, partially offsetting the higher cost of the drug. If, however, the baseline rates of angiography are different between countries, the cost implications of reducing angiography by one third in each country will be quite different (Table 6.5). A reduction by one third in the high rate of angiography in Country 1 (from 60% to 40%) provides a $200 cost offset per patient, whereas a reduction by one third in the low rate of angiography in Country 2 (from 20% to 15%) provides only a $50 cost offset per patient.

International comparisons of the cost of therapies can thus be affected by (a) differences in resource use patterns that reflect differences in practice style and the organization

Table 6.4 Effect of differences in medical prices on costs of alternative treatments

	Country 1			Country 2		
	Tx A		Tx B	Tx A		Tx B
Drug ($)	2000		200	1500		150
Nursing hours	50		54	50		54
Nursing wages ($)	30		30	35		35
Total ($)	3500		1820	3250		2040
Cost savings (A–B) ($)		1680			1210	
Cost ratio B/A		52%			63%	

Abbreviation: Tx, treatment

Table 6.5 Effect of differences in resource utilization on costs of alternative treatments

	Country 1			Country 2		
	Tx A		Tx B	Tx A		Tx B
Drug/nursing ($)	3500		1820	3250		2040
Coronary angiography	40%		60%	10%		15%
Angio cost ($)	1000		1000	1000		1000
Total ($)	3900		2420	3350		2190
Cost savings (A−B) ($)		1480			1160	
Cost ratio (B/A)		62%			65%	

Abbreviation: Tx, treatment

of medical care, and (b) by differences between countries in the prices attached to specific resources, such as healthcare wages, drugs, and supplies. Data from cost studies can be most readily applied in different practice environments if the study provides information on both resource consumption patterns and price weights attached to the specific resources used, as well as a summary cost measure. This detail is needed for readers to understand the applicability of the cost findings to their own practice settings.

Cost effectiveness analysis

The cost of providing a particular medical service can be measured, but determination of whether the service provides good value for the money spent is a more difficult judgment. Cost effectiveness analysis is a method of weighing the cost of a service in light of the health effects it confers in an attempt to facilitate the ultimate value judgment about whether the service is "worth" the cost.

Cost effectiveness analysis is one of several alternative analytic methods, each with its own strengths and limitations.[5] If two alternative therapies are either known to yield identical results or can be shown to be clinically equivalent, they can be compared on the basis of cost alone. This form of analysis, which is termed "cost-minimization analysis", is particularly appropriate to commodities such as drugs, supplies, and equipment that can be expected to yield equivalent results when applied clinically. In such situations, the relative costs of the alternatives become the predominant consideration.

Many alternative therapies are known to differ both in clinical outcomes and in cost. In this situation, both the difference in cost and the difference in effectiveness of the therapeutic alternatives must be measured and weighed against each other. When the effectiveness on intervention is measured in clinical terms (for example, lives saved, years of life added), the analysis is termed "cost effectiveness". If the clinical measures of effectiveness are translated into monetary units, the term "cost–benefit analysis" is applied.

Cost–benefit analysis has been used to guide public policy in areas outside of medicine, such as in the construction of transportation systems or whether to remove or reduce environmental exposures. Cost–benefit analysis measures the effects of programs in monetary terms, so that net cost (in dollars) can be compared with net benefits (in dollars). Since there is great reluctance on the part of physicians and health policy makers to assign a dollar value to saving a life or improving a patient's function, cost effectiveness analysis rather than cost–benefit analysis has been applied predominantly to medical problems.

Cost effectiveness analysis was first applied to medical programs only 25 years ago[8,9] and has since been widely used.[10–12] The principles of cost effectiveness analysis for medical programs have recently been examined in detail by a Task Force convened by the United States Public Health Service.[13–15] A group of experts attempted to establish consensus on a number of methodologic issues, with the goal of standardizing the technical aspects of cost effectiveness analysis among studies, thereby enhancing their comparability. The principles articulated by this group are reasonable, and should guide this important field in its next 20 years.

A basic principle of cost effectiveness analysis is that the analysis should compare alternative programs, and not look at any single program in isolation. Thus, a drug to treat life-threatening arrhythmias might be compared with placebo, or an implantable cardioverter defibrillator might be compared with a drug. In essence, cost effectiveness analysis must always answer the question "cost effective compared with what?".

Another principle is that the costs included in cost effectiveness analysis should be comprehensive. The cost of a specific therapy should include the cost of the intervention itself (for example, thrombolytic therapy for acute myocardial infarction) and the costs of any complications the therapy induced (for example, bleeding), less any cost savings due to reduction of complications (such as, heart failure). The need for other concomitant therapy should also be included, which is particularly important when assessing the cost effectiveness of screening programs or diagnostic testing strategies.

The length of follow up should be sufficient to include all relevant costs and benefits – such as readmissions to the hospital due to treatment failures. Non-monetary costs directly related to the medical intervention should also be included, such as the cost of home care by the patient's family, since omission of these costs would bias assessments toward programs that rely on unpaid work by family members or volunteers. Other costs not directly related to the intervention, however, such as the patient's lost wages or pension costs, are omitted by convention from the measured costs in a cost effectiveness analysis.

Another important issue in cost effectiveness analysis is the perspective taken by the analysis. There is general agreement that the analysis should include all relevant costs, regardless of who pays them. This principle is known as "taking the societal perspective", and it assures a complete accounting of costs in the analysis. A hospital, for instance, may not care about the out of pocket costs paid directly by the patient, but these are real costs and should be considered in the analysis.

Medical costs may accrue over long periods of time, especially in preventive programs or the treatment of chronic disease. Time scales of more than a year or so bring up two related but distinct issues – inflation and discounting. The nominal value of any currency changes over time; a dollar in 1977 had more purchasing power than a dollar in 1997. Studies conducted over long time periods will need to correct for the changing value of currencies, typically by application of the Consumer Price Index (or the GDP deflator). Application of the Consumer Price Index removes the effect of inflation, but does not address the separate issue of time preference for money. Even in a country free of inflation, citizens would prefer to receive $100 today than a promise they will be paid $100 in a year. One might have to promise to pay more money in a year, say $103, to compensate for the delay. The same is true in health programs: we would prefer to be paid today instead of in the future, and we would also prefer to pay our obligations in the future rather than today. Use of a discount rate provides a way to correct for the lower value of future costs relative to current costs. The technical experts' consensus is that future costs should be discounted at a rate equivalent to the interest paid on safe investments such as government bonds in an inflation-free environment, or about 3% per year. The effect of alternative discount rates between 0% and 5–10% per year should also be checked to document the sensitivity of the analysis to future costs.

In summary, a cost effectiveness analysis should include all medical costs, including those of complications of therapy and adverse effects prevented. The study should be of sufficient duration to measure all relevant costs and benefits of the treatment. All costs and benefits should be included, regardless of who bears or receives them. In studies covering more than a year or so, corrections should be made for inflation, and 3% per year discount rate should be applied to follow up costs.

Measuring effectiveness

The effectiveness of an intervention in practice can be measured in a variety of ways, with different outcome measures most appropriate for specific applications. Physiologic end points are often used in clinical trials, with the result of therapy assessed by a laboratory measure such as millimeters of mercury for blood pressure or episodes of non-sustained ventricular tachycardia on an electrocardiographic monitor. Laboratory measures are useful in judging the physiologic effects of therapy and its mechanism of action, but these surrogate markers may not predict the ultimate effect of therapy on mortality and morbidity, as vividly illustrated by the results of the Cardiac Arrhythmia Suppression Trial (CAST).[16] Physiologic end points are also tied closely to one specific disease, making comparisons against other benchmark therapies difficult. The patient and public are most concerned with the effect of therapy on survival and on their ability to function – that is, upon the length of life and the quality of life. A common denominator measure of effectiveness is thus the life years of expected survival, or the quality adjusted life years (QALYs). This measure is relevant to patients and to the public and can be applied to virtually any therapy.

Mortality is a common end point in clinical trials, and leads directly to the measure of life years of survival. The mean life expectancy of a cohort of patients is equal to the area under a standard survival curve. The difference in life expectancy between two therapies is therefore equal to the difference in the areas under their respective survival curves. Since many clinical studies do not follow patient cohorts long enough to observe complete survival times for all patients, some assumptions and modeling of long-term survival may be needed to estimate the full survival benefit of therapy for a cost effectiveness analysis.[17]

Improvement in quality of life is often as important to patients as reducing mortality, and it is often the main goal of therapies, such as the relief of disabling angina or improvement in exercise tolerance. A quality of life measure can be translated into a scale that ranges from a low of 0·0 (the worst possible health state, usually taken as death) to 1·0 (perfect health). This quality of life measure is multiplied by the length of time a patient spends in the health state to yield a quality adjusted life year (QALY). Thus:

$$\text{QALY} = \sum_{i} Q_i \times t_i$$

where QALY = the quality adjusted life years, Q_i = the quality factor for follow up period "i" and t_i = the length of time spent in period "i". This equation shows that the effectiveness of a treatment, as measured in QALYs, can be improved by either enhancing the patient's quality of life (Q_i) or the patient's length of life (t_i), or both.

Calculation of cost effectiveness

After the costs of therapy and the medical effectiveness of therapy have been assessed, cost effectiveness (CE) can be calculated as:

$$\text{CE ratio} = \frac{\text{Cost}_2 - \text{Cost}_1}{\text{QALY}_2 - \text{QALY}_1}$$

where Cost_1 and Cost_2 represent the costs of program 1 and program 2, respectively, and QALY_1 and QALY_2 represent the effectiveness of programs 1 and 2, respectively.

There are several implications of using this formula. First, cost effectiveness ratios that are positive (that is, >0) result if and only if one alternative has both higher cost and greater effectiveness – that is, $\text{Cost}_2 > \text{Cost}_1$ and $\text{QALY}_2 > \text{QALY}_1$ (or the reverse: $\text{Cost}_2 < \text{Cost}_1$ and $\text{QALY}_2 < \text{QALY}_1$). Cost effectiveness ratios of <0 are not generally important for decision making, since they arise only when one alternative has both lower costs and greater clinical effectiveness than the other (for example, $\text{Cost}_2 > \text{Cost}_1$, and $\text{QALY}_2 < \text{QALY}_1$). In this case, program 1 is superior in all respects: it has better outcomes and lower cost than program 2, and thus is said to "dominate" the alternative. The decision of which program to recommend is therefore simple.

Another important implication of the formula used to calculate cost effectiveness is that the ratio is undefined when the two alternatives provide equal outcomes, since when $\text{QALY}_2 = \text{QALY}_1$ the denominator in the cost effectiveness ratio is equal to zero. The implication is that when the difference in outcomes between two programs is negligible, cost effectiveness analysis is unnecessary, and the choice between two alternatives can be based on cost alone (that is, cost minimization analysis is more appropriate than cost effectiveness analysis).

Most commonly, one of two therapeutic alternatives has higher costs and greater effectiveness, and use of the formula yields a cost effectiveness ratio greater than zero. One treatment may have a cost effectiveness ratio of $5000 per year of life saved, and another might have a ratio of $75 000 per year of life saved. Since it is problematic to assign a dollar value to life, interpretation of these ratios is best made by consideration of benchmarks – other generally accepted therapies that serve as a rough gauge to an "acceptable" cost effectiveness ratio. Renal dialysis is a form of therapy that most people would consider expensive, and yet dialysis is an intervention that the USA and most other industrialized countries provide as a life saving therapy. The end stage renal disease program in the USA costs about $35 000 a year per patient, and if this therapy were withdrawn the patient would die. Thus, renal dialysis has a cost effectiveness ratio of $35 000 per year of life saved (or if one considers the reduced quality of life for a dialysis patient, perhaps $50 000 per quality adjusted year of life saved). Therapies with cost effectiveness ratios considerably more favorable than renal dialysis (that is, <$20 000) would be considered very cost effective, whereas therapies with cost effective ratios much higher (say >$75 000) would be considered too expensive.

Different societies may come to different conclusions about the level of cost effectiveness they consider good value. Wealthy countries with high per capita incomes are more willing to pay for expensive therapies than are poor countries. For instance, the percentage of gross domestic product and per capita health spending in Eastern Europe is much less than in Western Europe or North America, and these countries have not chosen to provide expensive services such as bypass surgery as readily or as frequently.

Decisions about funding programs might be more equitable and rational when guided by the relative cost effectiveness of programs. When studies use similar methods to measure cost and effectiveness, cost effectiveness ratios can be compared to rank the economic attractiveness of alternatives. Tables comparing various treatments, such as Table 6.6, have been termed "league tables" because of their similarity to the athletic league standings published in newspapers. Given the uncertainty inherent in measuring cost and effectiveness of medical interventions, and the methodologic variations among studies, only relatively large differences in cost effectiveness ratios should be considered significant. Thus, a program with a cost effectiveness ratio of $5000 per life year added is much better than one with a ratio of $30 000. Programs with ratios of $25 000 and $30 000 are so close that no firm conclusion about the relative values should be drawn.

Patient selection and cost effectiveness

Drugs and procedures in medicine are applied to different patient groups for different clinical indications. The medical effectiveness of therapies varies considerably according to patient selection. Cholesterol lowering therapy, for instance, will extend the life expectancy of a patient with multiple cardiac risk factors more than it will for a patient with the same cholesterol level and no other cardiac risk factors. Coronary bypass surgery provides greater life extension to a patient with left main coronary artery obstruction than it does to a patient with single vessel disease.[18] The cost effectiveness ratio for these therapies will therefore vary among patient subgroups due to the impact of patient characteristics on the clinical effectiveness of therapy, which forms the denominator of the cost effectiveness ratio. Similarly, the cost of a particular therapy may also vary according to patient characteristics, since the therapy itself may be more

Table 6.6 Cost effectiveness of selected cardiovascular therapies

Strategy	Patient group	Cost effectiveness[a]
Lovastatin	Post MI Men 45–54 Chol ≥ 250	Saves dollars and lives
Enalapril	CHF EF < 35%	Saves dollars and lives
Radio frequency ablation	WPW, post cardiac arrest	Saves dollars and lives
Physician counseling	Smoking	$1300
β blocker	Post-MI High-risk	$3600
CABG	Left main CAD Severe angina	$9200
β blocker	Post-MI Low-risk	$20 200
Lovastatin	Primary prevention Men 55–64 Chol > 300 Three risk factors	$20 200
tPA	Acute MI	$32 800
ICD	Sustained VT	$35 000
CABG	Two vessel CAD Angina	$42 500
Lovastatin	Primary prevention Men 55–64 Chol > 300 No other risk factors	$78 300
Exercise ECG	Asymptomatic 40 year old men	$124 400
CABG	Single vessel CAD Mild angina	$1 142 000
Lovastatin	Primary prevention 35–44 year old women Chol > 300 No other risk factors	$2 024 800

[a] $ values, dollars per year of life added.
Abbreviations: CAD, coronary artery disease; CHF, congestive heart failure; Chol, Cholesterol; ICD implantable defibrillator; MI, myocardial infarction; VT, ventricular tachycardia; WPW, Wolff–Parkinson–White syndrome; See glossary for other abbreviations
Source: adapted from Kupersmith *et al.*[10–12]

or less expensive according to different patient subgroups, or the likelihood of costly complications may be higher or lower in different groups of patients.

The clinical effectiveness of a therapy is generally the most important factor determining cost effectiveness. The reason for this importance is (a) that clinical effectiveness of a therapy generally varies more among patients than does the cost of therapy, and (b) the value of the cost effectiveness ratio is more sensitive to changes in the denominator (effectiveness) than to changes in numerator (cost). In the last analysis, a therapy must be clinically effective before it can be cost effective. Cost effectiveness analysis relies more on the assessment of medical effectiveness than it does on determination of cost.

Diagnostic tests and cost effectiveness

Cost effectiveness analysis has been applied primarily to assess specific therapies or therapeutic strategies, for which it is natural to measure effectiveness in terms of patient outcome. The principles of cost effectiveness can be extended to analyze screening tests and diagnostic strategies as well, but some additional factors must also be considered.

Therapies are expected to improve patient outcome *directly*, by intervening in the pathophysiology of disease processes. In contrast, a diagnostic test is expected to provide the physician with information about the patient, which in turn is expected to improve management and thereby *indirectly* improve patient outcome. The value of a test is therefore linked closely with patient selection for therapy, and the value of testing may well change as new therapies are developed, or alternative tests become available.

The information provided by a test may be used in different decisions, and the test may be more or less useful in these different settings. An exercise electrocardiogram, for example, can be used as a diagnostic test for coronary disease, a prognostic test for patients with recent myocardial infarction, a monitoring test to assess the effect of anti-ischemic therapy, or even as a way to establish target heart rates for an exercise training program. The efficacy and cost effectiveness of applying the exercise electrocardiogram will be different for these varied uses of the information provided by the test. The value of the test will depend on the indication for which it is used, much as the value of a β blocker will vary whether it is used to treat hypertension or as secondary prevention after a myocardial infarction.

The same test (for example, the exercise ECG) applied for the same purpose (such as diagnosis of coronary disease) will provide more information in some groups of patients than in others. As discussed elsewhere in this book, a diagnostic test provides more value if used when the pretest probability of disease is intermediate than when the pretest probability is either very high or very low. The test has the most value when the result is likely to change the estimated probability of disease such that clinical management is changed. Tests that never change patient management cannot change patient outcome, which is the "bottom line" in assessing cost effectiveness.

Conclusions

Economic analysis is designed to assist decisions about the allocation of scarce resources. Physicians now must address the cost implications of clinical decisions, and be aware of the effects on scarce resources. Economic efficiency is but one of many goals, however, and issues of fairness and humaneness are also central to medical care, and must be considered as well.

References

1. Fuchs VR. *Who shall live? Health, economics and social choice.* New York: Basic Books, 1974.
2. Jollis JG, Peterson ED, DeLong ER *et al.* The relation between the volume of coronary angioplasty procedures at hospitals treating Medicare beneficiaries and short-term mortality. *N Engl J Med* 1994;**331**:1625–9.
3. Kimmel SE, Berlin JA, Laskey WK. The relationship between coronary angioplasty procedure volume and major complications. *JAMA* 1995;**274**:1137–42.
4. Hannan EL, Racz M, Ryan TJ *et al.* Coronary angioplasty volume–outcome relationships for hospitals and cardiologists. *JAMA* 1997;**279**:892–8.
5. Drummond MF, Stoddart GL, Torrance GW. *Methods for the economic evaluation of health care programmes.* Oxford: Oxford University Press, 1987.
6. Finkler SA. The distinction between costs and charges. *Ann Intern Med* 1982;**96**:102–10.
7. Hlatky MA, Lipscomb J, Nelson C *et al.* Resource use and cost of initial coronary revascularization. Coronary angioplasty versus coronary bypass surgery. *Circulation* 1990;**82**(Suppl. IV): IV-208–IV-213.
8. Weinstein MC, Stason WB. Foundations of cost-effectiveness analysis for health and medical practices. *N Engl J Med* 1977;**296**:716–21.
9. Detsky AS, Naglie IG. A clinician's guide to cost-effectiveness analysis. *Ann Intern Med* 1990;**113**:147–54.
10. Kupersmith J, Holmes-Rovner M, Hogan A, Rovner D, Gardiner J. Cost-effectiveness analysis in heart disease, Part I: general principles. *Prog Cardiovasc Dis* 1994;**37**:161–84.
11. Kupersmith J, Holmes-Rovner M, Hogan A, Rovner D, Gardiner J. Cost effectiveness analysis in heart disease, Part II: preventive therapies. *Prog Cardiovasc Dis* 1995;**37**:243–71.
12. Kupersmith J, Holmes-Rovner M, Hogan A, Rovner D, Gardiner J. Cost effectiveness analysis in heart disease, Part III: ischemia, congestive heart failure, and arrhythmias. *Prog Cardiovasc Dis* 1995;**37**:307–46.
13. Russell LB, Gold MR, Siegel JE, Daniels N, Weinstein MC. The role of cost-effectiveness analysis in health and medicine. *JAMA* 1996;**276**:1172–7.
14. Weinstein MC, Siegel JE, Gold MR, Kamlet MS, Russell LB. Recommendations of the panel on cost effectiveness in health and medicine. *JAMA* 1996;**276**:1253–8.
15. Siegel JE, Weinstein MC, Russell LB, Gold MR. Recommendations for reporting cost-effectiveness analyses. *JAMA* 1996;**276**:1339–41.
16. Echt DS, Liebson PR, Mitchell LB *et al.* Mortality and morbidity in patients receiving encainide, flecainide, or placebo: the Cardiac Arrhythmia Suppression Trial. *N Engl J Med* 1991;**324**:781–8.
17. Mark DB, Hlatky MA, Califf RM *et al.* Cost effectiveness of thrombolytic therapy with tissue plasminogen activator as compared with streptokinase for acute myocardial infarction. *N Engl J Med* 1995;**332**:1418–24.
18. Yusuf S, Zucker D, Peduzzi P *et al.* Effect of coronary artery bypass graft surgery on survival: overview of 10-year results from randomized trials by the Coronary Artery Bypass Graft Surgery Trialists Collaboration. *Lancet* 1994;**344**:563–70.

7 Introduction to decision analysis

Kevin A Schulman, Henry A Glick, Allan S Detsky

The concept of evidence-based medicine challenges physicians to improve their use of the medical literature to guide their decision making in specific clinical settings. The concept is discussed extensively throughout this book. However, there are circumstances in which clinical trials do not address all of the issues of interest to a clinician. This may be because the trials do not compare the risks and benefits of all relevant treatment alternatives, or because the trials lack important data on the outcomes and costs of therapy. In these cases, researchers and clinicians are developing analytical strategies to improve their ability to synthesize the available information from the clinical literature and to help resolve these unanswered questions. One method of achieving this synthesis is the use of decision analysis, a set of mathematical strategies for aggregating information, making issues related to clinical decisions explicit, and solving for an optimal strategy under the constraints of the analysis. This decision analysis is a framework that can be used in the analysis of clinical problems as well as in economic analysis (see Chapter 6).

Decision analysis has been available to cardiologists for over 20 years.[1–3] In that time, the techniques have become more sophisticated and begun to address a broader range of questions.[4–6]

The goal of this chapter is to introduce the reader to some of the basic concepts of decision analysis and to review its use in the cardiovascular literature. For more specific information about the concepts or methods of decision analysis, the reader is referred to several excellent summary articles[2–11] or to one of the major texts in the field.[12–14]

Examples of decision analysis

In this section we present two examples of the use of decision analysis, a clinical example and an economic example. These are provided to demonstrate the steps involved in developing a decision analysis. As will be clearly demonstrated, decision analytic models must simplify reality in order to structure the problem and analysis. Although our examples are extremely simplified to illustrate the steps involved in decision analysis, many models in the clinical literature offer more complex depictions of clinical reality.[16–22,26,27,36,40,41,53–58]

Steps in decision analysis

1. Identify the strategic options.
2. Draw the tree (structure of outcomes).
3. Determine the probabilities.
4. Determine the relevant outcome measures (effects, utility, survival, costs).
5. Evaluate the tree.
6. Make a structured analysis of the problem.
7. Develop a conclusion.

A comparative clinical analysis: warfarin *v* aspirin for atrial fibrillation

For patients with non-valvular atrial fibrillation, both warfarin and aspirin have been shown to reduce the risk of stroke.[28–35] However, the effectiveness and side effects of these two treatments can vary substantially. As there has been no randomized trial of aspirin and warfarin for stroke prevention, decision analysis has been used to identify the clinical outcomes resulting from treatment with each medication.[36]

Step 1: Identify the strategic options

In terms of therapeutic benefit, patients who receive either warfarin or aspirin experience a reduction in the risk of stroke. However, patients receiving these therapies also experience risk of bleeding complications. Both stroke and hemorrhage can be either fatal or non-fatal.

Step 2: Draw the tree

Based on these facts, we can graphically depict the issue using a decision tree (Figure 7.1). The tree is displayed so that the decision of interest is on the left side of the diagram, while the strategies to be compared are in the center, and the outcomes of those strategies are on the right. There are several pieces of information included in this simple figure.

In the decision tree a choice is represented by a square, also called a "decision node". In this example, the decision node represents a choice between warfarin and aspirin. Once a decision is made, patients experience the potential

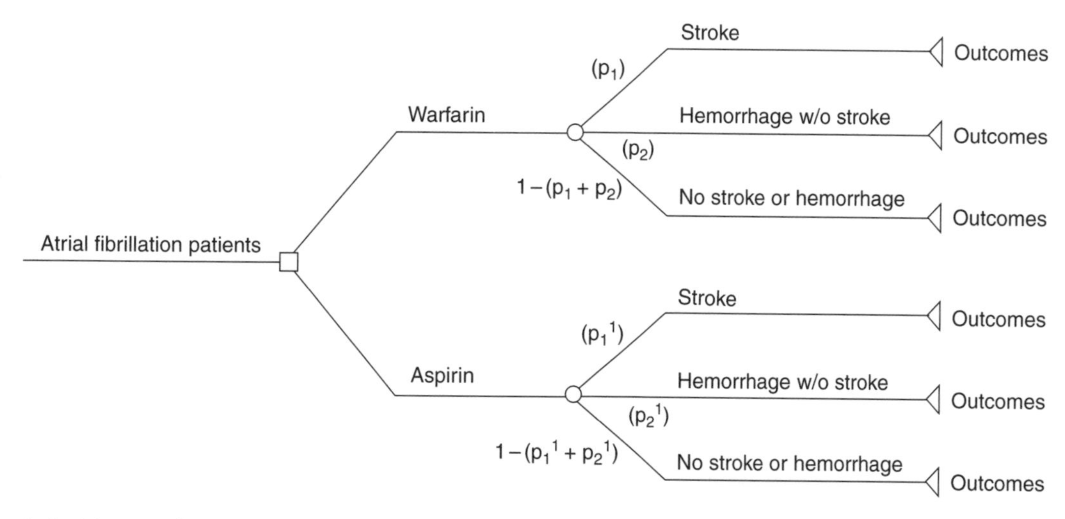

Figure 7.1 A decision tree for a comparative clinical analysis: warfarin *v* aspirin for atrial fibrillation

for different clinical events (stroke or hemorrhage). These decisions and their subsequent clinical events are represented by lines or "pathways" running through the tree diagram. Figure 7.1 contains six possible pathways: warfarin with stroke; warfarin with neither stroke nor hemorrhage; warfarin with hemorrhage but without stroke; aspirin with stroke; aspirin with neither stroke nor hemorrhage; and aspirin with hemorrhage but without stroke.

After the initial treatment decision between warfarin and aspirin has been made, subsequent outcomes occur with a defined probability such that all of the potential treatment outcomes are represented by the treatment pathways. The individual patient's achievement of a given treatment outcome (for example stroke or no stroke) is not a decision: it is, instead, a chance occurrence, where the "chance" event is represented by a circle in the decision tree.

The final treatment outcomes for each pathway are represented by triangles. These figures represent the outcomes of each treatment strategy. One, two or more outcomes can be expressed for each pathway (survival, quality adjusted survival, or costs).

Step 3: Determine the probabilities

Once a tree has been developed to depict a clinical problem, the next step is to begin to develop the data required to complete the analysis. In our example, we must identify the probability of stroke for patients in our two treatment categories and identify the potential risk of bleeding complications associated with each therapy.

Rates of stroke without therapy, outcomes of stroke, and stroke risk reduction with prophylaxis with aspirin or warfarin can be estimated from clinical trials or epidemiologic studies.[36] Rates of major hemorrhage associated with warfarin and aspirin therapy, and the outcomes of such an event, can be estimated in the same fashion.[36] However, in pooling these various data sources, investigators are left with a degree of uncertainty about these estimates. Sensitivity analysis, a method for assessing the impact of uncertainty in data analysis of clinical problems, will be discussed later, but it is an integral component of most well constructed decision analytic models.

Step 4: Determine the relevant outcome measures (effects, utility, survival, costs)

For this analysis, quality adjusted survival will be the primary outcome measure. Other possible outcome measures include event-free survival or simple survival. Analysis of quality adjusted survival uses estimates of patient preferences for a variety of possible health states for patients with stroke. Patient preferences are a measure of health-related quality of life, or utility, as defined on a 0–1 scale, in which 0·0 represents the worst imaginable health state and 1·0 denotes the best imaginable health state. Quality adjusted survival is the product of the expected survival of patients and their preferences for the different health states resulting from a stroke or hemorrhage. These data can be estimated from expert opinion, as reported in the medical literature, or derived from patient interviews.[37] Calculation of quality adjusted life years (QALYs) is described in greater detail elsewhere.[9]

Step 5: Evaluate the tree

Once data have been compiled for the specified model parameters, the next step is to analyze the tree. This requires the calculation of the expected value for each pathway of the tree. For both warfarin and aspirin therapies, the expected value of the outcome (effects, utility, survival or costs) is a weighted average of all possible treatment outcomes. This weighted average is calculated as the product of the value of each terminal node and the probabilities of the occurrence of that node (the product of the probabilities of achieving that node). The value of each node is then summed to result in the weighted average value for the treatment (for example, the outcome for warfarin would be the weighted average of the products of the probability of stroke while taking warfarin and the outcome for stroke ($P1 \times O1$), the probability of hemorrhage without stroke while taking warfarin and the outcome for hemorrhage without stroke ($P2 \times O2$), and the probability of no stroke or hemorrhage and the outcome for no stroke or hemorrhage $\{(1 - [P1 + P2]) \times O3\}$).

A more complicated decision analysis proceeds in stepwise fashion for each set of probabilities and outcomes. This is called folding back the tree. The net result is an assessment of the outcomes for the two treatments, warfarin and aspirin. Other techniques can be used to solve more complicated problems, for which there are many branches of each tree – for example, when the risk of stroke or hemorrhage is related to the duration of treatment. (These methods are based on the probability of moving between health states over time. Analysis can also be based on "state transition models" or Markov models.)

For clinical analyses, decision trees allow an incremental analysis of the treatment benefits of one medical therapy compared to another. They are used to compare the expected utility for each branch of the tree to pick the best treatment option. The best option is the one with the highest value in terms of clinical effects (survival or utility) or the one with the smallest value in terms of cost. An incremental analysis assesses the additional benefits gained from one treatment and, thus, differs from a calculation of the absolute benefit of a treatment.

Step 6: Structured analysis of the problem

Finally, the primary analysis having been completed, investigators should examine uncertainty in their estimates using a technique called sensitivity analysis. By recognizing that a decision tree can suffer from uncertainty in the probability of each treatment strategy, investigators can ask how the results might change were the possibilities of stroke or hemorrhage to increase or decrease by 10% for each treatment arm. In a sensitivity analysis, the investigator recalculates the results of the model to address the robustness of the analysis to changes in the model specification.

Step 7: Conclusion

This decision analysis was structured to compare the outcomes of two strategies for the treatment of stroke prophylaxis – warfarin and aspirin. Such an analysis allows for an assessment of the clinical benefits of the two strategies, incorporating both the differences in risk reduction of stroke and the differences in hemorrhage resulting from the prophylactic treatment. The analysis would end with an estimate of the quality adjusted survival resulting from each treatment strategy. The results could reveal that warfarin is superior to aspirin, that aspirin is superior to warfarin, that the treatments are comparable, or that there is not enough information from which to draw a firm conclusion. The analysis would also address how sensitive the analysis was to differing model parameters. This could help define areas for further research to resolve outstanding issues in the clinical assessment.

A cost effectiveness analysis: implantable cardiac defibrillators

At present there is a great deal of debate about the most appropriate treatment of patients with arrhythmias, especially about whether implantable cardiac defibrillators (ICDs) will reduce cost and mortality for high-risk patients. Early clinical trial results address mortality issues related to the use of ICDs in high-risk populations.[38] However, there remains a great deal of concern about the findings of the study and the robustness of its results.[39] Although decision analysis cannot answer the clinical questions regarding ICD use, these techniques have been used to model the costs and effects of ICD insertion to estimate the potential cost effectiveness of this therapy, given current estimates of ICD clinical effectiveness.[40,41] To understand the decision analysis approach to this question, we will review the clinical issues and then build a decision analytic model to formalize the question.

High-risk patients experience an increased incidence of sudden cardiac death.[42] One new technology, the ICD, has been proposed as a means of reducing the incidence of sudden death in cardiac patients.[38,43–48] Patients who choose to receive this therapy must undergo a surgical procedure and maintain the device over the remainder of their lifetime.

Step 1: Identify the strategic options

In terms of treatment benefit, patients who receive an ICD have the potential for a different survival probability than patients who do not receive an ICD. From a cost perspective, patients receiving an ICD bear the additional cost of the device itself, as well as the future costs of maintaining it.

Step 2: Draw the tree

Based on this discussion, we can graphically depict the issue using a decision tree (Figure 7.2). There are four possible pathways in this figure: ICD with sudden death; ICD without sudden death; no ICD with sudden death; and no ICD without sudden death. In this simple model we consider only two health states: sudden death and no sudden death.

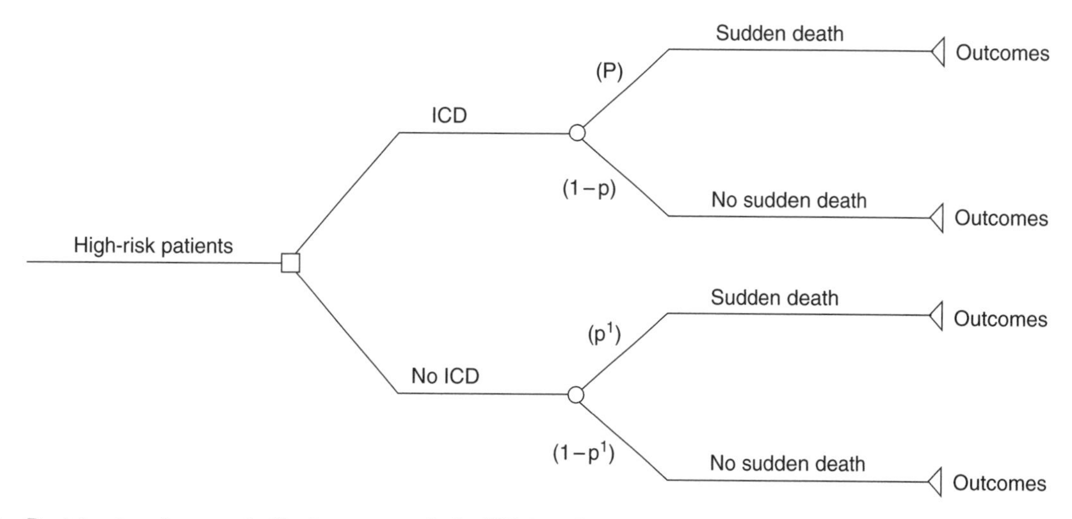

Figure 7.2 Decision tree for a cost effectiveness analysis: ICD to reduce incidence of sudden death in cardiac patients

Step 3: Determine the probabilities

Estimates of the possibility of sudden cardiac death for high-risk patients are available in the medical literature and in trials of ICDs.[43–49] Estimates of the probability of sudden death for patients receiving an ICD are available from the MADIT Study[38] or may be estimated based on clinical trial protocols for expected treatment benefits.[41] The quality of the evidence from these data sources can vary. Data from the literature on non-ICD patients, the probability of sudden death without an ICD, come from observational studies, whereas data on ICD patients come from a controversial randomized controlled trial. Thus, there is some uncertainty about these estimates.[10]

Step 4: Determine the relevant outcome measures (effects, utility, survival, costs)

Treatment benefits can be expressed in terms of survival (years of life gained) or in terms of quality adjusted survival (QALYs). Calculation of these benefits proceeds as outlined in the stroke example.

Estimates of treatment costs often must be developed from primary sources (for example, hospital accounting departments), from standard price lists for specific costs,[50] from literature reviews, or from expert opinion. Costs included in these models can include direct medical costs (the costs of medical care, such as hospital or physician costs), direct non-medical costs (the costs patients incur in receiving medical care services, such as the cost of transportation to a physician's office), indirect costs (the costs of morbidity or mortality related to disease), or intangible costs (the costs of pain and suffering related to disease).[51,52]

Step 5: Evaluate the tree

Once the data are available for all of these model parameters, the next step is to analyze the tree. For economic analyses, decision trees allow an incremental analysis of the treatment costs and benefits of one medical therapy compared to another in a cost effectiveness analysis. The incremental cost effectiveness of therapy A compared to therapy B is defined by the following formula:

$$\text{Cost effectiveness of treatment A} = \frac{(\text{Cost}_A - \text{Cost}_B)}{(\text{Effects}_A - \text{Effects}_B)}$$

where Cost_A is the cost of treatment A, Cost_B is the cost of treatment B, Effects_A are the effects of treatment A, and Effects_B are the effects of treatment B.[52] Decision trees may also allow enumeration of the costs and consequences of different treatments without comparing the costs and effects of treatment in a cost effectiveness ratio.

Step 6: Structured analysis of the problem

Sensitivity analysis would be conducted to assess the impact of uncertain values on the model. For example, because there was uncertainty in the probability of each treatment strategy, how would the results change if the possibilities of sudden death were increased or decreased by 10% for each treatment arm? Similarly, how would the results differ if ICD costs were increased or decreased by 10%? In a sensitivity analysis, the investigator recalculates the results of the model to address the robustness of the analysis to changes in the model specification.

Step 7: Conclusion

This decision analysis was structured to assess the cost effectiveness of a new therapy for the treatment of patients at high risk for sudden cardiac death. It would conclude with an estimate of the incremental effects of ICD therapy in years of life gained per patient, the incremental costs of ICD treatment per patient, and an estimate of the cost effectiveness of

ICD therapy for patients evaluated in the model. The paper would also address how sensitive the analysis was to different model parameters. This sensitivity analysis could help define areas for further research to resolve outstanding issues in the clinical assessment.

Applications of decision analysis to cardiology

The above examples offer a simplified explanation of some of the basic components of decision analysis. They also illustrate the issues that must be addressed before using the results of a decision analysis to guide clinical decision making. As when reviewing clinical trials, clinicians must assess whether the population considered in the decision analysis model is relevant to their own population. The reader must consider the strength of the evidence available to the investigator in developing the model to understand the strength of the recommendations resulting from the model. This includes not only whether the evidence was based on randomized controlled trials or on observational studies, but also whether the original studies included detailed information required by the model (for example, in the stroke analysis, whether the clinical studies reported both hemorrhage and stroke rates for the study's patients). Finally, the reader should consider the model used by the investigator to determine whether it was constructed appropriately and considered all relevant comparisons.[1,5] The models below that use lower-quality data or evidence should be considered exploratory analyses, not definitive evidence. As such, they also should be interpreted as potential rationale for future studies. Likewise, decision models that project results to new time periods, new populations and new interventions – even those that use A1a-grade evidence – should be viewed only as exploratory analyses.

Decision analysis has been used extensively in cardiology over the past several years (Table 7.1). These examples include articles from a MEDLINE search of decision analysis and cardiology from 1993 to 2001. Issues addressed have included the use of specific technologies, such as ICDs for patients at risk for sudden death, as well as specific diagnostic or pharmacologic products for defined populations of patients (for example, treatment of high blood cholesterol), and the assessment of patient management strategies for defined populations of patients (for example the selection of patients for placement on a cardiac transplant list). Each of the analyses listed in Table 7.1 will be reviewed in this section.

Table 7.1 Use of decision analysis in the cardiovascular literature

Clinical issue	Efficacy data	Cost data	Sensitivity analysis	Source	Evidence grade*
New technologies					
Inpatient ICD placement	Observational study; utility not assessed	Hospital charges; literature review for resource use data	Yes	Kupersmith *et al*[16]	B4
Outpatient ICD placement	Literature review for survival and utility estimates	Hospital and claims data; literature review for resource use data	Yes	Owens *et al*[41]	A1c
Treatment strategies for WPW syndrome	Literature review; expert opinion; authors' estimates for utility data	Cost-accounting data for 13 patients at one study center	Yes	Hogenhuis *et al*[17]	B4
Specific products					
Low *v* high-osmolality contrast media	Literature review; authors' estimates for utility data; patient survey for intangible cost estimates	Resource use from a clinical trial; literature review; costs from Canadian hospital	Yes	Barrett *et al*[18]	A1c
Simvastatin, high cholesterol	Clinical trial data; utility not assessed	Resource use from clinical trial; costs from hospitals in Sweden; employment status from clinical trial	Yes	Johannesson *et al*[19]	A1a

Table 7.1 *Continued*

Clinical issue	Efficacy data	Cost data	Sensitivity analysis	Source	Evidence grade*
Pravastatin, high cholesterol	Clinical trial data from 2 studies; utility not assessed	Literature review and expert opinion for resource use data; costs from aggregate US hospital data	Yes	Ashraf *et al*[20]	A1c
Captopril, acute MI	Clinical trial data; utility data from 82 patients	Resource use from subset of study patients; costs from US Medicare reimbursement rates	Yes	Tsevat *et al*[21]	A1a
Estrogen replacement	Literature review; utility not assessed	Not assessed	Yes	Zubialde *et al*[22]	B2
Streptokinase *v* tPA, suspected MI	Literature review, including utility data	Resource use estimated; drug and hospital cost data from Ireland	Yes	Kellett *et al*[26]	A1a
Warfarin *v* quinidine *v* amiodarone, acute atrial fibrillation	Literature review and expert opinion, including utility data	Not assessed	Yes	Disch *et al*[27]	A1a
Warfarin *v* aspirin, stroke prophylaxis	Literature review; utility data from study of 74 patients	Resource use estimated; costs from literature review, Medicare data, and survey of pharmacies	Yes	Gage *et al*[36]	A1a
Preoperative coronary angiography and revascularization, non-cardiac vascular surgery	Literature review; utility not assessed	Literature review	Yes	Mason *et al*[55]	A1a
Treatment strategies					
CCU admission	Cohort study; utility not assessed	Hospital charges from the cohort adjusted to costs	Yes	Tosteson *et al*[56]	B4
Emergency medical services	Literature review; utility not assessed	Analysis of existing EMS program in Canada	Yes	Nichol *et al*[57]	B4
Cardiac transplantation selection	Transplant registries	Not assessed	Yes	Stevenson *et al*[58]	B4
Aortic valve replacement				Wong *et al*[59]	B4
Medical *v* surgical therapy for chronic stable angina	Expert guidelines, randomized trials, and meta-analyses; utility not assessed	Not assessed	Yes	Kwok *et al*[61]	A1a
Strategies for hypoplastic left heart syndrome	Literature review and data from 231 patients; utility not assessed	Not assessed	Yes	Jenkins *et al*[62]	B3

Table 7.1 ***Continued***

Clinical issue	Efficacy data	Cost data	Sensitivity analysis	Source	Evidence grade*
Electrocardiogram algorithm to predict myocardial infarction	Retrospective cohort study; utility not assessed	Not assessed	Yes	Shlipak *et al*[63]	B2

*Evidence grades for decision analysis are complicated by the many different sources of data used in constructing the analysis. Evidence grades here are based on the data for the most important component of the analysis for the clinical portion of the decision tree. Where sources of evidence for the analysis were from a variety of sources, two grades were assigned to reflect the differing quality of data available for the analysis (see Owens *et al.*[41] for an example of grades of evidence for data incorporated into a decision analysis).
Grade A: Decision trees with the primary effect estimate from a large, high-quality study (a randomized controlled trial with more than 500 patients), or decision trees with a formal meta-analysis for the primary effect estimate.
Grade B: Decision trees with the primary effect estimate based on literature review but without a formal meta-analysis for primary effect estimate; includes evidence from case series and randomized controlled trials with fewer than 500 patients.
Grade C: Decision trees with the primary effect estimate based on expert opinion.

Decision analysis evaluating new technologies

ICD placement

Over the past several years, investigators have attempted to calculate the cost effectiveness of the ICD in patients at high risk for sudden cardiac death. Recent evidence from the Antiarrhythmics versus Implantable Defibrillators Trial indicates a decrease of 27% in 2 year mortality with ICD.[15] Kupersmith *et al*[16] assessed ICD placement on an inpatient basis for patients with and without prior electrophysiologic (EP) studies. **Grade A1c** The investigators assumed an 84% improvement in life expectancy for patients undergoing ICD therapy based on a case series of 218 non-randomized patients who received an ICD when it was assumed that the patients would have died at the time of the first event (first shock or death). In this analysis, ICD patients had a mean life expectancy of 3·78 years, whereas EP-guided drug therapy patients had a mean life expectancy of 2·06 years. Total charges for these treatments were $146 797 for ICD patients and $93 340 for the EP-guided patients. The investigators found that the cost of ICD placement, including the cost of the device and the hospitalization, would range between $27 200 and $44 000 per year of life saved.

The investigators conducted an extensive sensitivity analysis around their cost data and around the period of replacement of the ICD generator. They found that the cost effectiveness of the therapy was sensitive to the magnitude of the clinical benefit of the therapy (this included the efficacy of the therapy, as well as the estimated life expectancy for the underlying population, as represented by ejection fraction). The model was less sensitive to the cost of ICD therapy. The authors concluded that ICD use was economically attractive, especially using endocardial lead placement (based on preliminary estimates of the cost of this new procedure).*

Owens *et al*[41] assessed ICD implantation on an outpatient basis using a decision analytic model. In this analysis, the investigators modeled the potential cost effectiveness of therapy, assuming in their principal analysis that the ICD led to a 20–40% reduction in mortality. **Grade A1c** The investigators found that the cost of patients receiving ICD therapy would be $88 400, and the cost of patients receiving amiodarone therapy alone would be $51 000. For high-risk

* There are four possible outcomes of a cost effectiveness analysis: (1) the intervention will save money and be more effective than the comparison; (2) the intervention will cost money and be more effective than the comparison; (3) the intervention will save money and be less effective than the comparison; and (4) the intervention will cost money and be less effective than the comparison.[51] The first outcome is the most preferred, and the intervention will always be adopted. The last outcome is never preferred, and the intervention will never be adopted. The second and third outcomes may be preferred at times, and the interventions may be adopted, depending on the relationship between the costs and effects of the intervention (the cost effectiveness ratio). The second outcome may be adopted if the intervention yields a great enough benefit for the additional cost (in the USA, an economically attractive intervention may be one that costs less than $50 000 per year of life gained, whereas some Canadian authors have suggested that therapies that cost less than CDN$100 000 might be economically attractive).[35,53] The third outcome may be adopted if the intervention yields a small enough reduction in outcomes for the reduction in cost (for example, the same Canadian authors suggested an economically attractive intervention might be one that saves more than CDN$100 000 per year of life forgone).[35,52]

patients, the investigators reported that ICD patients would have an estimated survival of 4·18 QALYs, whereas patients treated with amiodarone alone could expect a survival of 3·68 QALYs. Investigators found that the cost effectiveness of therapy ranged from $37 300 per QALY saved for high-risk patients, assuming a 40% reduction in mortality for patients treated with the ICD compared to those treated with amiodarone alone, to $138 900 QALYs saved for intermediate-risk patients and assuming a 20% reduction in mortality for patients treated with the ICD compared to amiodarone alone. They concluded that the use of an ICD will not be economically attractive unless all-cause mortality is reduced by 30% or more compared to amiodarone.

Alternative therapies for WPW syndrome

Hogenhuis *et al*[17] determined which of five management strategies should be used for the treatment of patients with Wolff–Parkinson–White (WPW) syndrome: observation, observation until cardiac arrest-driven therapy, initial drug therapy guided by non-invasive monitoring, initial radiofrequency ablation, and initial surgical ablation. The model included the risks of cardiac arrest, arrhythmia, drug adverse effects, procedure-related complications and mortality, and assumed that radiofrequency ablation had an overall efficacy of 92% in preventing cardiac arrest and arrhythmia. **Grade B4**

For survivors of a cardiac arrest, radiofrequency ablation offered additional survival at reduced cost compared to all other treatment strategies. For patients with arrhythmia without hemodynamic compromise, radiofrequency ablation resulted in a cost of $6 600 per QALY gained in 20 year old patients and $19 000 per QALY gained in 60 year old patients without hemodynamic compromise. For asymptomatic patients, radiofrequency ablation costs from $33 000 per QALY gained in 20 year old patients to $540 000 per QALY gained for 60 year old patients. The authors conclude that their analysis supports the practice of radiofrequency ablation in patients with WPW syndrome who survive cardiac arrest. For asymptomatic patients, however, the analysis supports the current practice of mere observation, given that radiofrequency ablation was economically unattractive in this population of patients.

Decision analysis in the evaluation of specific products

Decision analysis has been used extensively in the evaluation of specific clinical products, including contrast media and pharmaceutical products.

Contrast media

Grade A1c Barrett *et al*[18] developed a decision analytic model to assess the economic impact of low- and high-osmolality contrast media for cardiac angiography. Investigators assumed that low-osmolality contrast media reduced the risk of myocardial infarction and stroke. Reduction in the risk of specific clinical events with low-osmolality contrast media was assumed to be 0% in fatal events, 25% in severe events, 80% in moderate events and 10% in minor events. The investigators found that the incremental cost per QALY gained with these media was $17 264 in high-risk patients and $47 874 in low-risk patients for a third-party payer. From a societal perspective, the corresponding costs are $649 and $35 509. The authors report that these estimates were sensitive to cost of the contrast media and the total cost of contrast media used per patient. The authors also suggest that the model is extremely sensitive to changes in assumptions regarding the efficacy of low-osmolality contrast media for the prevention of severe reactions. To allow the reader to better understand the inputs of this model, the authors include a cost–consequence analysis of the program as a separate presentation in the results. The authors concluded that, in the context of restricted budgets, limiting the use of low-osmolality contrast media to high-risk patients is justifiable. The recommendation to limit use of this medium was also justified by the lack of clinical evidence that low-osmolality contrast media prevent severe or fatal reactions.

Cholesterol reduction

Several authors have used decision analysis to investigate the cost effectiveness of therapies designed to reduce high blood cholesterol.[54] Two recent studies use clinical trial data to assess the cost effectiveness of cholesterol reduction in secondary prevention of coronary artery disease. Johanneson *et al*[19] developed an analysis based on the Scandinavian Simvastatin Survival Study, which reported that, in patients with pre-existing coronary disease, reduction in blood cholesterol resulted in a 30% reduction in overall mortality based on a median follow-up of 5·4 years. **Grade A1a** The authors modeled the effects of 5 years of cholesterol-reducing therapy on patients' outcomes, using a model based on data reported from the trial. The costs of therapy were based on the assumption that the use of cholesterol-reducing agents would not entail any additional costs for patients with pre-existing coronary disease other than the cost of medication itself, and then used data on hospitalizations to estimate the direct medical costs incurred for the treatment of cardiovascular disease.

Interestingly, this model also included the indirect costs of medical care based on the employment status of patients in the trial. The investigators found that simvastatin treatment for 5 years in 59 year old patients with a history of heart disease and a pretreatment total cholesterol level of 261 mg/dl would have a net cost of $1 524, with 0·28 years of life gained, resulting in a cost per year of life gained of $5 400 for men, and a net cost of $1 685 with 0·61 years of life gained, resulting in a cost per year of life gained of $10 500 for women. An analysis that included direct and indirect costs showed that cholesterol reduction leads to an additional $1 065 decrease in associated morbidity cost for men and an $876 reduction in associated morbidity cost for women. The analysis was somewhat sensitive to baseline cholesterol level and patient age at the initiation of treatment, to follow-up and screening costs and to the price of simvastatin. However, treatment remained economically attractive in all of these analyses. The model was somewhat sensitive to reduction in cardiovascular risk and the risk of mortality after coronary events. The authors concluded that in patients with coronary artery disease, simvastatin therapy is economically attractive among both men and women at the ages and cholesterol levels studied.

Ashraf *et al*[20] assessed the cost effectiveness of cholesterol reduction based on 3 year data from the Pravastatin Limitation of Atherosclerosis in the Coronary Arteries (PLAC I) and Pravastatin, Lipids and Atherosclerosis in the Carotids (PLAC II) studies. **Grade A1c** These trials reported no statistically significant decrease in all-cause mortality, but did report a decrease in the number of coronary events in men in the group receiving drug therapy to reduce high blood cholesterol. Therapy was estimated using a Markov model based on data from the Framingham Heart Study to estimate subsequent annual morbidity and mortality rates for patients with non-fatal myocardial infarction. Costs of therapy were based on the costs of drug therapy, and hospitalization costs were derived from the cost of treatment of myocardial infarction and from expert opinion on the frequency of medical events. Investigators found that cost per year of life saved due to secondary prevention was sensitive to a number of risk factors, but ranged from $7124 per year of life saved for a male patient with three risk factors, to $12 665 per year of life saved for a male patient with one risk factor. The model was sensitive to assumptions about efficacy of therapy and cost of services. It was also sensitive to patient characteristics, such as the number of risk factors of patients receiving secondary prevention. The authors conclude that pravastatin is economically attractive compared to other widely accepted medical interventions.

A potentially serious limitation of the Ashraf *et al*[20] analysis is its strategy of deriving costs for 3 years while projecting the effects over 10 years. Specifically, the authors project years of life saved by avoiding events in the first 3 years over the next 7 years. This potentially problematic practice of generating a differential time horizon should be avoided.

Postmyocardial infarction treatment

Tsevat *et al*[21] used decision analysis to assess the cost effectiveness of captopril therapy after acute myocardial infarction (MI). **Grade A1a** In this paper, the investigators used data from the Survival and Ventricular Enlargement (SAVE) trial, which demonstrated that captopril therapy reduced mortality in patients who survived MI. The effectiveness of therapy was modeled using a decision analytic model based on all-cause mortality within the clinical trial observation period and the projected clinical benefits over a patient's lifetime. This paper also incorporated data on quality of life from a subset of patients in the SAVE trial. Cost estimates for the model were based on a subset of 123 study patients for whom hospital data were obtained for all hospitalizations in the subset. The investigators used two projection methods, a limited-benefit model and a persistent-benefit model. The limited-benefit model was more conservative in that it assumed similar annual mortality rates between captopril and control patients beyond the clinical trial period. This analysis resulted in an estimated cost effectiveness for captopril therapy ranging from $60 800 per QALY for 50 year old patients to $3 600 per QALY for 80 year old patients. The persistent-benefit model was more optimistic in that it assumed that the clinical benefits observed in the trial persisted throughout each patient's lifetime. In this analysis, the cost effectiveness ratios were similar to those in the limited-benefit model for patients aged 60–80 years, but they were substantially better for 50 year old patients. In the sensitivity analysis, the models were most sensitive to the annual cost of captopril therapy. In addition, the persistent-benefit model appeared to be more "stable" than the limited-benefit analysis. That is, when the benefits persist, there are few changes to the values of other variables that would affect the resulting cost effectiveness ratios (owing to the magnitude of the benefit), whereas if the benefits do not persist, variations in other variables do have an effect. The investigators concluded that angiotensin converting enzyme inhibitor therapy with captopril was not only effective in improving survival after MI, but also moderately economically attractive.

Hormone replacement therapy

Zubialde *et al*[22] used a decision analytic model to assess gains in life expectancy resulting from the use of estrogen replacement therapy for postmenopausal women. Efficacy data for this analysis were obtained from a review of the literature which suggested that risk reduction with estrogen therapy for coronary artery disease was between 40% and 50%. **Grade B2** The model did not assume an increased incidence in breast cancer in the principal analysis, but it did include an increased incidence of endometrial cancer. Results of the analysis suggested that the benefit of estrogen and progesterone therapy in average-risk women aged 50 years at the time of therapy initiation was 0·86 years, with a range of 0·41–1·19 years, whereas therapy in average-risk women aged 65 years at the time of therapy initiation was 0·47 years, with a range of 0·21–0·66 years. The authors reported that the benefits of estrogen and progesterone therapy were similar to the gains from cholesterol reduction to

200 mg/dl and smoking cessation. The authors concluded that significant potential benefits in life expectancy in coronary artery disease reduction, combined with the osteoporosis prevention in symptom relief, would point to greater emphasis on postmenopausal estrogen use in appropriate patients. Since the report by Zubialde *et al*[22] hormone replacement therapy has undergone additional study. A growing body of literature suggests that its predicted effects have not been fully realized,[23,24] and the results of a recent polymorphism study have further complicated matters.[25] It bears repeating here that the reliability of a decision analysis is related directly to the quality of the data on which the analysis is based. The Zubialde analysis was based on the best data of its time, but superior data from clinical trials have since called the findings into question.

Thrombolytic therapy

Kellett *et al*[26] presented a paper on the use of thrombolytic therapy for patients with suspected MI. This assessed the use of two types of thrombolytic therapy, streptokinase and accelerated tissue plasminogen activator (tPA), on patients with suspected MI. **Grade A1a** The efficacy of the two therapies was based on reports from the medical literature. The authors assessed the clinical benefits of thrombolytic therapies for patients presenting with different likelihoods of MI, given their clinical and ECG findings, different age groups, and different probabilities of death given MI. Data on clinical efficacy for the two strategies were based on the GISSI-2, ISIS-3 and GUSTO trials. The authors suggested that, for patients with a 26% probability of MI (a group with chest pain and a history of coronary artery disease but a normal ECG), thrombolytic therapy would only be beneficial if the probability of death given an MI was 20% or greater. In contrast, for patients presenting with a probability of MI of 78% (chest pain plus ST or T wave changes), thrombolytic therapy would be beneficial for all patients except those over 80 years of age who had a probability of death given an MI of 2·5% or less. The authors conclude that, for a typical 60 year old man presenting 4 hours after the onset of symptoms with definite acute MI, treatment with streptokinase in addition to aspirin would gain 150 quality adjusted life days, whereas treatment with aspirin and accelerated tPA would result in 255 quality adjusted life days, compared to no thrombolytic therapy. Thrombolytic therapy is preferred over no thrombolytic therapy as long as the probability of stroke is less than 5% for streptokinase and 8% for accelerated tPA. The cost per QALY was estimated based on the probability of acute MI, the extra days of quality adjusted life, and the probability of death given an MI. The analysis was sensitive to estimates of efficacy for both streptokinase and accelerated tPA, as well as the probability of death given thrombolytic therapy. The authors conclude that decision analysis can be a useful bedside tool to guide thrombolytic therapy. It is important to bear in mind, however, that this decision model has not been tested on actual patients.

Management of atrial fibrillation

Dirsch *et al*[27] developed a decision analytic model to assess the outcomes of four treatment strategies for patients with acute atrial fibrillation undergoing cardioversion: warfarin therapy, quinidine therapy and low-dose amiodarone therapy. **Grade A1a** Efficacy was based on a review of the literature, including randomized controlled trials, observational studies, and expert clinical opinion when necessary. Investigators found that all four treatment strategies differed by 0·2 QALYs over patients' lifetimes, with 4·55 expected QALYs for patients who undergo no treatment after cardioversion and 4·75 expected QALYs for patients who undergo cardioversion with amiodarone. Use of warfarin and quinidine therapies yielded expected quality adjusted life benefits between amiodarone and no treatment. The model was sensitive to the annual rate of bleeding on warfarin, the annual rate of stroke for patients on warfarin, the annual rate of stroke for patients with atrial fibrillation, the decrement in quality of life associated with taking warfarin, and the excess mortality of quinidine and amiodarone. The authors conclude that cardioversion followed by low-dose amiodarone to maintain normal sinus rhythm appears to be a relatively safe and effective treatment for a hypothetical cohort of patients with atrial fibrillation.

Prophylaxis of stroke

Gage *et al*[36] developed a decision analytic model to assess the cost effectiveness of warfarin and aspirin treatment for prophylaxis of stroke in patients with non-valvular atrial fibrillation. The clinical efficacy of the treatment strategies was obtained from the published literature. **Grade A1a** The quality-of-life estimates for this study were obtained by interviewing patients with atrial fibrillation. Costs were also estimated from a literature review and from a survey of national pharmacies and laboratories. The authors found that, for patients with non-valvular atrial fibrillation and no additional risk factors for stroke, warfarin would minimally affect quality adjusted survival but increase costs significantly. For patients with non-valvular atrial fibrillation and one additional risk factor, warfarin therapy resulted in a cost of $8 000 per QALY saved compared to aspirin. The model was most sensitive to the rate of stroke if no therapy was prescribed, the effectiveness of aspirin, the rates of major hemorrhage, and the disutility of taking warfarin. The authors conclude that treatment with warfarin is economically attractive (has a low cost effectiveness ratio) in patients with non-valvular atrial fibrillation and one or more additional risk factors for stroke. However, in patients with non-valvular atrial fibrillation without other risk factors for stroke, the use of warfarin instead of aspirin would add significantly to costs with minimal additional clinical benefit.

Preoperative cardiac revascularization

Mason *et al*[55] developed an analysis to determine whether preoperative coronary angiography and revascularization improved short-term outcomes in patients undergoing non-cardiac vascular surgery with three strategies. **Grade A1a** The first was to proceed directly to vascular surgery; the second was to perform coronary angiography followed by selective coronary revascularization prior to surgery and to cancel vascular surgery in patients with severe inoperable coronary disease; and the third was to perform coronary angiography followed by selective coronary revascularization, and to perform vascular surgery in patients with inoperable coronary artery disease. The literature was scrutinized for data on the efficacy of all three strategies. The authors found that proceeding directly to vascular surgery led to a lower morbidity and cost in the base-case analysis. The coronary angiography strategy led to a higher mortality of vascular surgery in patients with inoperable coronary disease, but to a lower mortality in operable patients who did not proceed to vascular surgery. The model was sensitive to the surgical mortality rates for both catheterization and the vascular surgical procedure. The authors concluded that decision analysis indicates that vascular surgery without preoperative angiography generally leads to better outcomes, and that preoperative coronary angiography should be reserved for patients whose estimated mortality for vascular surgery is substantially higher than average.

Use of decision analysis in treatment strategies

CCU admission

Tosteson *et al*[56] used a decision analytic model to identify cost effective guidelines for admission to a coronary care unit (CCU) for uncomplicated patients without other indications for intensive care. The probabilities of death, and minor, major and life-threatening complications were based on 12 139 emergency department patients who were enrolled in a multicenter chest pain study. Cost data were available from a subset of patients in the study admitted to one study center. Under the assumption that there is a 15% relative increase in mortality when patients with acute MI are admitted to the intermediate care unit instead of an intensive CCU, the authors found that costs per year of life saved for triage to the CCU varied markedly depending on the age of the patient and the probability of MI. For 55–64 year old patients with an emergency department probability of infarction of 1%, the cost per year of life saved was $1·4 million; but when the probability of infarction was 99%, the cost per year of life saved was $15 000. Admission to the intensive care unit was generally more costly for younger patients, and use of the CCU had a cost effectiveness ratio of less than $50 000 per year of life saved when the initial probability of acute MI was greater than 57% among patients 30–44 years of age, and greater than 21% among patients 65–74 years of age. The model was sensitive to the reduction of mortality associated with the use of the intensive care unit and to the costs of the intensive care unit. The authors conclude that the CCU should generally be reserved for patients with a moderate or high probability of acute MI, unless they need intensive care for other reasons.

Emergency medical services

Nichol *et al*[57] used a decision analytic model to assess the cost effectiveness of potential improvements to emergency medical services (EMS) for patients with out-of-hospital cardiac arrest. **Grade B4** The authors developed their analysis based on a review of the effectiveness of various emergency systems from an extensive meta-analysis, costing of each component of the EMS, and community characteristics and response times for EMS. The authors also modeled a one-tier system versus a two-tier system. In the one-tier system the response team is trained in advanced life support, and in the two-tier system the first response team is trained in basic life support and the second in advanced life support. The authors found that the fixed cost of the first tier of a two-tier EMS system was $651 129 for Hamilton, Ontario, with estimates of survival of 5·2% in the one-tier system and 10·5% in the two-tier system. They found that a 1 minute reduction in response time improved survival by 0·4% in a one-tier system and by 0·7% in a two-tier system. The authors found that a change from a one-tier system to a two-tier system would result in 0·19 QALYs saved and an incremental cost of $7 700 per patient, or a cost per QALY of $40 000. Improvement in a one-tier EMS system by the addition of more basic life support providers in the first tier would result in an incremental survival benefit of 0·40 QALYs, with an incremental cost of $2 400 or cost per QALY of $53 000. An improvement in response time in a one-tier system by the addition of more providers and ambulances would achieve an incremental survival benefit of 0·2 QALYs for a cost per QALY of $368 000. The authors performed an extensive sensitivity analysis based on a combination of the model's parameters. They concluded that the most attractive options in terms of incremental cost effectiveness ratios for an EMS program would be improved response time in a two-tier EMS system, or a change from a one-tier EMS system to a two-tier system. However, the authors were concerned about the poor quality of the data available for their analysis.

Heart transplantation

Stevenson *et al*[58] used a decision analytic model to determine optimal strategies for selecting patients for cardiac transplantation. **Grade B4** The authors developed a model based on data from cardiac transplantation databases. The decision analytic model was developed to determine the size and outcomes of the waiting list population, depending upon different strategies for listing heart transplant candidates. They found that if current practices continued all hearts would be transplanted to hospitalized candidates and newly listed urgent candidates, and 3700 outpatient transplant candidates would be listed with virtually no transplantation unless they deteriorated to an urgent status. A decrease in the upper age limit for transplantation to 55 years would reduce the number listed each month by 30%. If this strategy were to be adopted, the waiting list would reduce to one third its current size, with 50% of all hearts being available for outpatient candidates. The authors conclude that immediate provisions should be made to limit candidate listing and revise expectations to reflect the diminishing likelihood of transplantation for outpatient candidates.

Surgery for aortic stenosis

Wong *et al*[59] used decision analysis to assess whether to recommend cardiac surgery for elderly women with aortic stenosis. **Grade B4** This analysis was based on a specific case of assessing the treatment choice for an 87 year old patient with severe aortic stenosis, three vessel coronary disease, depressed left ventricular function and moderately severe heart failure. Data for the analysis were based on the medical literature. Specific data elements included in the analysis were life expectancy with and without surgery for an octogenarian, morbidity and mortality associated with surgery, and quality of life with congestive heart failure. Sensitivity analysis assessed the sensitivity of the model to assumptions used in developing the analysis and assessed the impact of patients' risk preferences regarding treatment choice. The authors also modeled valvuloplasty compared to surgery. They found that life expectancy with surgery (5·0 QALYs) was greater than that for medical therapy (1·1 QALYs). (These gains in life expectancy are substantial. Most interventions reported in the medical literature yield incremental gains in life expectancy from 0·167 to 1·2 years of life.[60]) In sensitivity analysis, surgery still had the highest life expectancy until mortality from the procedure was greater than 70%. Valvuloplasty was the best strategy if the patient was not the best candidate for surgery or, perhaps, in cases in which the perioperative mortality rate was greater than 50%. They concluded that even in the later decades of life, aortic valve surgery is substantially preferable to medical therapy.

Treatment strategies for chronic stable angina

Kwok *et al*[61] used a decision analytic model to simulate a randomized controlled trial of coronary artery bypass graft surgery versus medical therapy for chronic stable angina. **Grade A1a** The authors developed a Markov model that incorporated current American College of Cardiology/ American Heart Association guidelines, baseline data from a meta-analysis of randomized trials of the two therapies, and risk reduction data from randomized trials and meta-analyses. The outcome measures of interest were 5 and 10 year mortality, as well as incidence of non-fatal myocardial infarction. The authors conducted a base-case analysis of the two therapies, which they supplemented with annual fixed transition probabilities to account for a steady linear increase in mortality observed in the meta-analysis. They also conducted two subgroup analyses, one to examine 5 year mortality and infarction rates for patients with triple vessel disease, the other to examine the same outcomes for patients with impaired left ventricular function. In the base-case and subgroup analyses, the authors found that both therapies increased overall and infarction-free survival. The relative advantage of surgery over medical therapy found in this study mirrored the findings of previous trials. One-way and multiway sensitivity analyses yielded absolute differences of less than 2% for overall and infarction-free survival rates, except that use of the upper limit of aspirin therapy's relative reduction of myocardial infarction yielded a 3% increase in infarction-free survival among patients receiving medical therapy. The authors concluded that therapeutic advances have improved outcomes for both medical and surgical patients, as well as preserving the advantages of surgery, thereby confirming that the conclusions of previous bypass trials remain valid.

Treatment strategies for hypoplastic left heart syndrome

Jenkins *et al*[62] used a decision analytic model to determine the optimal treatment strategy for maximizing 1 year survival among patients with hypoplastic left heart syndrome. **Grade B3** Using data from the literature and from a data set of 231 patients treated at four US surgical centers, the authors obtained probabilities for the following treatment strategies: complete staged surgery; stage 1 surgery as an interim to transplantation; patient listing, then stage 1 surgery if no donor is found within 1, 2 or 3 months; and patient listing without surgery until transplantation. The authors conducted one- and two-way sensitivity analyses on all probabilities in the decision tree to determine the values at which the optimal treatment strategy would change. In the base-case analysis, transplantation within 1 month emerged as the preferred strategy, followed by staged surgery if no donor is available after listing the patient for 1 month. These results were sensitive to several probability thresholds, including stage 1 and stage 2 mortality rates, the surgical center's 3 month organ donation rate, and the transplantation mortality rate. Centers with high organ donation rates are best served by a strategy of listing without surgery until transplantation. Those with low donation rates, however, should perform staged surgery. In two-way sensitivity analyses, the authors found that the highest 1 year survival rates were achieved with staged surgery; patient listing, then stage 1 surgery at 1 month; and listing without surgery until transplantation. The authors concluded that each surgical center can determine its optimal treatment strategy with an algorithm that uses the center's organ donation rates and stage 1 survival outcomes, as well as individual patients' risk factors for mortality and organ availability.

Use of electrocardiogram to predict myocardial infarction

Shlipak *et al*[63] used a decision analytic model to assess the clinical utility of a previously reported electrocardiogram (ECG)-based algorithm to predict myocardial infarction in patients with left bundle branch block (LBBB). **Grade B2** The authors developed probability data for their analysis by first conducting a retrospective cohort study of patients presenting with LBBB on their initial ECG. The subsequent decision analysis was performed to determine which of the following strategies would constitute optimal therapy: thrombolysis for all patients with LBBB; no treatment for these patients; or use of the ECG-based algorithm to screen patients for the appropriateness of thrombolysis. The authors found that the ECG algorithm had low sensitivity and would predict less than 10% of myocardial infarctions in patients presenting with LBBB and acute symptoms. As a screening test, the algorithm resulted in a survival rate less than that yielded by thrombolysis and similar to that yielded by no therapy. In one-way sensitivity analysis, thrombolysis was always the optimal strategy. In two-way sensitivity analyses thrombolysis was always preferred, unless the ECG-based algorithm had a sensitivity greater than 85%. If the ECG algorithm were used as a screening test for thrombolytic therapy, almost no patients with LBBB and myocardial infarction would receive the treatment. The authors conclude that the ECG algorithm is a poor predictor of myocardial infarction and that thrombolysis should be used for all patients with LBBB and symptoms of myocardial infarction.

Summary

Decision analysis offers powerful techniques to better understand uncertain clinical decisions in cardiology. Increasing use of these techniques has already shown them to be very valuable in clinical and policy decision making in a variety of settings. Decision analysis may be most useful when clinical trial data do not clearly answer the clinical issue; when the clinical trial concludes that there are differences in risks and benefits across two treatment groups; when the relevant outcomes were not collected as part of the clinical trial; or when the decision maker is concerned with both clinical benefits and costs. Readers of a decision analysis paper should consider the strength of the evidence underlying the analysis, whether the model was constructed appropriately from a clinical perspective, and whether all relevant comparisons were included in the model.[5,6]

Key points

- Decision analysis may be most useful when clinical trial data do not clearly answer the clinical issue; when the clinical trial concludes that there are differences in risks and benefits across two treatment groups; when the relevant outcomes were not collected as part of the clinical trial; or when the decision maker is concerned with both clinical benefits and costs.
- Sensitivity analysis is used to assess the impact of uncertainty on decision analytic models.
- In reviewing a decision analysis paper, the reader must assess whether the population considered in the model is relevant to the clinician's population, the strength of the evidence available to the investigator in developing the model, and whether the model used by the investigator is constructed appropriately by including all relevant comparisons.
- Decision analysis has been used to assess a wide variety of clinical issues in cardiology.

Acknowledgment

The authors are grateful to Damon Seils for research and editorial assistance.

References

1.Paulker SA. Coronary artery surgery: the use of decision analysis. *Ann Intern Med* 1976;**85**:8–18.
2.Detsky AS, Naglie G, Krahn MD, Naimark D, Redelmeier DA. Primer on medical decision analysis: Part 1 – getting started. *Med Decis Making* 1997;**17**:123–5.
3.Stason WB, Weinstein MC. Allocation of resources to manage hypertension. *N Engl J Med* 1977;**296**:732–9.
4.Kassirer JP, Moskowitz AJ, Lau J, Pauker SG. Decision analysis: a progress report. *Ann Intern Med* 1987;**106**:275–91.
5.Richardson WS, Detsky AS. User's guide to the medical literature: VII. How to use a clinical decision analysis: A. Are the results of the study valid? *JAMA* 1995;**273**:1292–5.
6.Richardson WS, Detsky AS. User's guide to the medical literature: VII. How to use a clinical decision analysis: B. What are the results and will they help me in caring for my patients? *JAMA* 1995;**273**:1610–13.
7.Greenberg ML, Malenka DJ, Disch DL. Therapeutic strategies for atrial fibrillation: the value of decision analysis. *Cardiol Clin* 1996;**14**:623–40.

8. Detsky AS, Naglie G, Krahn MD, Redelmeier DA, Naimark D. Primer on medical decision analysis: Part 2 – building a tree. *Med Decis Making* 1997;**17**:126–35.
9. Naglie G, Krahn MD, Naimark D, Redelmeier DA, Detsky AS. Primer on medical decision analysis: Part 3 – estimating probabilities and utilities. *Med Decis Making* 1997;**17**: 136–41.
10. Krahn MD, Naglie G, Naimark D, Redelmeier DA, Detsky AS. Primer on medical decision analysis: Part 4 – analyzing the model and interpreting the results. *Med Decis Making* 1997;**17**:142–51.
11. Naimark D, Krahn MD, Naglie G, Redelmeier DA, Detsky AS. Primer on medical decision analysis: Part 5 – working with Markov processes. *Med Decis Making* 1997;**17**:152–9.
12. Weinstein MC, Fineberg HV *et al. Clinical decision analysis.* Philadelphia: WB Saunders, 1980.
13. Sox HC, Blatt MA, Higgins MC, Marton KI. *Medical decision making.* Boston: Butterworth–Heinemann, 1988.
14. Petitti DB, Sidney S, Quesenberry CP Jr, Bernstein A. Incidence of stroke and myocardial infarction in women of reproductive age. *Stroke* 1997;**28**:280–3.
15. The Antiarrhythmics versus Implantable Defibrillators (AVID) Investigators. A comparison of antiarrhythmic-drug therapy with implantable defibrillators in patients resuscitated from near-fatal ventricular arrhythmias. *N Engl J Med* 1997;**337**: 1576–83.
16. Kupersmith J, Hogan A, Guerrero P *et al.* Evaluating and improving the cost-effectiveness of the implantable cardioverter-defibrillator. *Am Heart J* 1995;**130**:507–15.
17. Hogenhuis W, Stevens SK, Wang P *et al.* Cost-effectiveness of radiofrequency ablation compared with other strategies in Wolff–Parkinson–White syndrome. *Circulation* 1993;**88**: 437–46.
18. Barrett BJ, Parfrey PS, Foley RN, Detsky AS. An economic analysis of strategies for the use of contrast media for diagnostic cardiac catheterization. *Med Decis Making* 1994;**14**: 325–35.
19. Johannesson M, Jönsson B, Kjekshus J *et al.* Cost-effectiveness of simvastatin treatment to lower cholesterol levels in patients with coronary heart disease. *N Engl J Med* 1997;**336**:332–6.
20. Ashraf T, Hay JW, Pitt B *et al.* Cost-effectiveness of pravastatin in secondary prevention of coronary artery disease. *Am J Cardiol* 1996;**78**:409–14.
21. Tsevat J, Duke D, Goldman L *et al.* Cost-effectiveness of captopril therapy after myocardial infarction. *J Am Coll Cardiol* 1995;**26**:914–19.
22. Zubialde JP, Lawler F, Clemenson N. Estimated gains in life expectancy with use of postmenopausal estrogen therapy: a decision analysis. *J Fam Pract* 1993;**36**:271–80.
23. Hulley S, Grady D, Bush T *et al.* Randomized trial of estrogen plus progestin for secondary prevention of coronary heart disease in postmenopausal women. *JAMA* 1998;**280**:605–13.
24. Herrington DM, Reboussin DM, Brosnihan KB *et al.* Effects of estrogen replacement on the progression of coronary-artery atherosclerosis. *N Engl J Med* 2000;**343**:522–9.
25. Herrington DM, Howard TD, Hawkins GA *et al.* Estrogen-receptor polymorphisms and effects of estrogen replacement on high-density lipoprotein cholesterol in women with coronary disease. *N Engl J Med* 2002;**346**:967–74.
26. Kellett J, Clarke J. Comparison of accelerated tissue plasminogen activator with streptokinase for treatment of suspected myocardial infarction. *Med Decis Making* 1995;**15**:297–310.
27. Dirsch DL, Greenberg ML, Holzberger PT, Malenka DJ, Birkmeyer J. Managing chronic atrial fibrillation: a Markov decision analysis comparing warfarin, quinidine, and low-dose amiodarone. *Ann Intern Med* 1994;**120**:449–57.
28. The European Atrial Fibrillation Trial Study Group. Secondary prevention in non-rheumatic atrial fibrillation after transient ischæmic attack or minor stroke. *Lancet* 1993;**342**:1255–62.
29. Connolly SJ. Canadian Atrial Fibrillation Anticoagulation (CAFA) Study. *J Am Coll Cardiol* 1991;**18**:349–55.
30. Ezekowitz MD, Bridgers SL, James KE *et al.* Warfarin in the prevention of stroke associated with nonrheumatic atrial fibrillation. *N Engl J Med* 1992;**327**:1406–12.
31. Stroke Prevention in Atrial Fibrillation Investigators. Stroke Prevention in Atrial Fibrillation (SPAF) Study: final results. *Circulation* 1991;**84**:527–39.
32. Stroke Prevention in Atrial Fibrillation Investigators. Warfarin versus aspirin for prevention of thromboembolism in atrial fibrillation: Stoke Prevention in Atrial Fibrillation II Study. *Lancet* 1994;**343**:687–91.
33. Petersen P, Boysen G, Godtfredsen J, Andersen ED, Andersen B. Placebo-controlled, randomised trial of warfarin and aspirin for prevention of thromboembolic complications in chronic atrial fibrillation: the Copenhagen aFASAK Study. *Lancet* 1989; **i**:175–9.
34. The Boston Area Anticoagulation Trial for Atrial Fibrillation Investigators. The effect of low-dose warfarin on the risk of stroke in patients with nonrheumatic atrial fibrillation. *N Engl J Med* 1990;**323**:1505–11.
35. Laupacis A, Feeny D, Detsky AS, Tugwell PX. How attractive does a new technology have to be to warrant adoption and utilization? Tentative guidelines for using clinical and economic evaluations. *Can Med Assoc J* 1992;**146**:473–81.
36. Gage BF, Cardinalli AB, Albers GW, Owens DK. Cost-effectiveness of warfarin and aspirin for prophylaxis of stroke in patients with nonvalvular atrial fibrillation. *JAMA* 1995;**274**: 1839–45.
37. Solomon NA, Glick HA, Russo CJ, Schulman KA. Patient preferences for stroke outcomes. *Stroke* 1994;**25**:1721–5.
38. Moss AJ, Jackson Hall W, Cannom DS for the Multicenter Automatic Defibrillator Implantation Trial (MADIT) Investigators. Improved survival with an implanted defibrillator in patients with coronary disease at high risk for ventricular arrhythmia. *N Engl J Med* 1996;**335**:1933–40.
39. Friedman PL, Stevenson WG. Unsustained ventricular tachycardia – to treat or not to treat? *N Engl J Med* 1996; **335**:1984–5.
40. Boyko W, Schulman KA, Tracy CM, Glick H, Solomon AJ. The economic impact of prophylactic defibrillators. *J Am Coll Cardiol* 1997;**29**(2 Suppl A):256A.
41. Owens DK, Sanders GD, Harris RA *et al.* Cost-effectiveness of implantable cardioverter defibrillators relative to amiodarone for prevention of sudden cardiac death. *Ann Intern Med* 1997;**126**:1–12.
42. Schatzkin A, Cupples LA, Heeren T *et al.* The epidemiology of sudden unexpected death: risk factors for men and women in the Framingham Heart Study. *Am Heart J* 1984;**107**:1300–6.

43. Pinski SL, Trohman RG. Implantable cardioverter-defibrillators: implications for the nonelectrophysiologist. *Ann Intern Med* 1995;**122**:770–7.
44. The Coronary Artery Bypass Graft (CABG) Patch Trial Investigators and Coordinators. The CABG Patch Trial. *Prog Cardiovasc Dis* 1993;**36**:97–114.
45. Cardiomyopathy Trial Investigators. The cardiomyopathy trial. *Pacing Clin Electrophysiol* 1993;**16**:576–81.
46. The DEFIBRILAT Study Group. Actuarial risk of sudden death while awaiting cardiac transplantation in patients with atherosclerotic heart disease. *Am J Cardiol* 1991;**68**:545–6.
47. AVID Trial Investigators. Antiarrhythmics Versus Implantable Defibrillators (AVID) – rationale, design, and methods. *Am J Cardiol* 1995;**75**:470–5.
48. Connolly SJ, Gent M, Roberts RS *et al.* Canadian Implantable Defibrillator Study (CIDS): study design and organization. *Am J Cardiol* 1993;**72**:103F–8F.
49. Hine LK, Laird NM, Hewitt P, Chalmers TC. Meta-analysis of empirical long-term antiarrhythmic therapy after myocardial infarction. *JAMA* 1989;**262**:3037–40.
50. Health Care Financing Administration. Revisions to payment policies and adjustments to the relative value units under the physician fee schedule for calendar year 1995; Final rule. *Fed Reg* 2 December 1995.
51. Eisenberg JM, Schulman KA, Glick H, Koffer H. Pharmacoeconomics: economic evaluation of pharmaceuticals. In: Strom BL, ed. *Pharmacoepidemiology*, 2nd edn. New York: John Wiley & Sons, 1994.
52. Detsky AS, Naglie IG. A clinician's guide to cost-effectiveness analysis. *Ann Intern Med* 1990;**113**:147–54.
53. Naimark DM, Detsky AS. The meaning of life expectancy: what is a clinically significant gain? *J Gen Intern Med* 1994;**9**:702–7.
54. Glick H, Heyse JF, Thompson D *et al.* A model for evaluating the cost-effectiveness of cholesterol-lowering treatment. *Int J Technol Assessment Hlth Care* 1992;**8**:719–34.
55. Mason JJ, Owens DK, Harris RA, Cooke JP, Hlatky MA. The role of coronary angiography and coronary revascularization before noncardiac vascular surgery. *JAMA* 1995;**273**:1919–25.
56. Tosteson ANA, Goldman L, Udvarhelyi S, Lee TH. Cost-effectiveness of a coronary care unit versus an intermediate care unit for emergency department patients with chest pain. *Circulation* 1996;**94**:143–50.
57. Nichol G, Laupacis A, Stiell IG *et al.* Cost-effectiveness analysis of potential improvements to emergency medical services for victims of out-of-hospital cardiac arrest. *Ann Emerg Med* 1996;**27**:711–20.
58. Stevenson LW, Warner SL, Steimle AE *et al.* The impending crisis awaiting cardiac transplantation: modeling a solution based on selection. *Circulation* 1994;**89**:450–7.
59. Wong JB, Salem DN, Paulke SG. You're never too old. *N Engl J Med* 1993;**328**:971–5.
60. Naimark DM, Detsky AS. The meaning of life expectancy: what is a clinically significant gain? *Med Decis Making* 1992;**12**:344.
61. Kwok YS, Kim C, Heidenreich PA. Medical therapy or coronary artery bypass graft surgery for chronic stable angina: an update using decision analysis. *Am J Med* 2001;**111**:89–95.
62. Jenkins PC, Flanagan MF, Sargent JD *et al.* A comparison of treatment strategies for hypoplastic left heart syndrome using decision analysis. *J Am Coll Cardiol* 2001;**38**:1181–7.
63. Shlipak MG, Lyons WL, Go AS *et al.* Should the electrocardiogram be used to guide therapy for patients with left bundle-branch block and suspected myocardial infarction. *JAMA* 1999;**281**:714–9.

8 Assessing and changing cardiovascular clinical practices

C David Naylor, David A Alter

Research into cardiovascular clinical practice has grown early enormously in volume and sophistication since the early twentieth century, driven by the worldwide prominence of atherosclerotic vascular diseases. The sheer volume of research literature has made it virtually impossible for even a subspecialist to stay abreast of her/his field. There is insufficient time for any evidence-oriented practitioner to critically appraise the full array of individual studies relevant to practice, and a real risk that, as the years go by, his/her filtering of the literature will prove misleading.

One solution is for practitioners to rely increasingly on integrative reports. As documented throughout this volume, evidence on a particular clinical topic is often usefully compiled in published meta-analyses, decision analyses, or practice guidelines. These integrative reports synthesize the best evidence available from multiple research studies to help define what a practitioner ought to do when confronted with a particular clinical situation.

While information uptake from integrative reports is necessary to ensure that clinical care evolves in evidence-driven directions, it may not be sufficient. For decades, researchers have shown that the rates of provision of various cardiovascular services vary inexplicably across regions and among nations. Some of this variation is random; some represents reasonable disagreement in the absence of definitive evidence about best practices. However, when practices are examined more closely using explicit criteria for appropriateness of care, it has become clear that actual practice sometimes differs sharply from what the evidence suggests ought to be done, raising concerns about quality of care. Quality concerns are further galvanized by evidence that technical skill and patient outcomes vary among procedural specialists. Not surprisingly, then, concerns with costs and quality of care have led a growing cadre of researchers, clinical leaders, facility managers, third party payers, and public policy makers to examine what clinicians do, and to seek ways to change clinical practice.

Assessing and changing clinical practice is central to the discipline commonly known as health services research. This chapter accordingly provides an introduction to some of the key methods of health services research as applied to cardiovascular medicine and surgery.

By definition this chapter demands a different treatment than later chapters where it is possible to provide integrative summaries of evidence to inform contemporary practice or steer future research. Since our focus is on how evidence is translated into clinical action, it stands to reason that there will seldom be one "right answer". Practice will instead be shaped not just by evidence, but by values and circumstances or context. Thus, it is important for the reader to suspend judgment as to whether there is necessarily one right health system, or one right profile of services for all populations with a given cardiovascular condition. A corollary of this point is that hundreds of descriptive and analytical studies have been published in cardiovascular health services research, many of which are context-specific. Our hope is to use a small number of these studies to heighten the reader's understanding of analytical principles and general lessons. For consistency, the examples will relate to clinical management of coronary artery disease, not to primary and secondary prevention. However, the conceptual frameworks are applicable to all areas of cardiovascular care. It is hoped that the evidence-oriented reader will be able to generalize the methodological insights from this chapter to his/her particular clinical and research context.

The specific objectives of this chapter are three:

- to outline the challenges and opportunities in gathering evidence about how health care is delivered;
- to describe and provide illustrations of the various types of studies done to evaluate processes and outcomes of care; and
- to examine some of the interventions that can be undertaken to improve the quality of cardiovascular care.

Gathering evidence about health care: challenges and opportunities

Study designs

Randomized controlled clinical trials are the most rigorous tool for confirming causal relationships between a given outcome and intervention or factor. Most randomized clinical trials are designed to test the efficacy of an intervention within a controlled and stable environment. In contrast, health services research focuses on assessing and improving the provision of care in usual practice settings. Observational studies of health services may be cross-sectional or cohort designs. Cross-sectional studies or survey designs offer convenient one-off snapshots of patient populations, providers, or practice settings. Disease- and procedure-specific inception cohorts have the advantage of delineating relationships of particular variables to outcomes over time.

Cross-sectional and cohort methodologies can also be combined in a single study. For example, Payne and Saul[1] undertook a mail survey of a random sample of 16 750 residents of the Sheffield (UK) region, and found that 4·0% of subjects had symptoms suggestive of angina pectoris. The prevalence of angina was significantly higher in neighborhoods with lower socioeconomic status, but these same areas had significantly lower rates of mechanical revascularization. In other words, variations in service profiles were inversely related to ecological markers of both population need and population deprivation – obvious grounds for concern about access or equity of services use. The authors went further, however, and used data linkage methods to determine procedures that were actually provided to individuals identified as having angina. In so doing, they effectively shifted from a cross-sectional study reliant on ecological inferences to a full-fledged cohort design. They found that among subjects reporting angina who lived in affluent neighborhoods, 11·2% had undergone procedures, as compared to 4·2% in less affluent areas ($P=0{\cdot}03$). Similar socioeconomic-related disparities in cardiovascular processes of care have been well described in both private and publicly-funded healthcare systems.[2,3]

Intervention studies in health services research focus on effectiveness and efficiency rather than efficacy. Quasi-experimental designs and formal randomized clinical trials are brought into play to test interventions designed to improve care. However, for obvious reasons, it is often providers, clinics, hospitals, or regions that are randomized rather than patients.[4]

Whatever the internal validity of the design chosen, health services researchers face a recurrent challenge to prove the external validity of their work. Some of the published literature in health services research consists of local or regional quality assurance projects with uncertain generalizability, and evidence-oriented practitioners may not find these studies applicable in their own context.

Data sources and collection

Health services researchers use both primary and secondary data sources. *Primary data* are collected by design to answer specific research questions, whereas *secondary data* are used for multiple purposes and their use for research purposes may be unplanned. Administrative databases designed for purposes of health service funding and administration are among the most common secondary data sources used in assessing clinical practice. Databases specifically constructed for ongoing epidemiologic surveillance of medical care, such as clinical registries, sit on the cusp between primary and secondary data, in that they are valuable for management and quality assurance, but are usually designed to meet specific research objectives as well.

Prospective primary data collection is costly but crucial for complex variables that are poorly covered in most secondary data sources – for example, patients' quality of life and psychosocial status. Retrospective primary data collection through chart reviews is also possible, but can be costly and time-consuming. It is best focused on routinely-recorded variables. For example, in charts of patients hospitalized with acute myocardial infarction (AMI), data on variables such as presenting symptoms, heart rate, blood pressure, ECGs, and cardiac enzymes are almost uniformly recorded. Absent primary data collection, there is always a risk that researchers will frame their questions around convenient access to data rather than addressing pressing issues.

Researchers often combine primary and secondary data collection, or incorporate multiple data sources to address specific research questions. For instance, a study may assess patients' short-term outcomes using self-administered health status questionnaires, and then track their subsequent use of health services and outcomes through administrative data. As an inexpensive solution to the limitations of single secondary databases, many researchers now link data across multiple administrative databases to provide better patient characterization and longitudinal follow up.[5] Finally, linkage of samples from randomized clinical trials to administrative databases is becoming more common both to provide accurate and cost efficient follow up of clinical trial populations and to enable comparison of the characteristics and outcomes of trial participants to the broader populations from which they are drawn.[6]

Data quality

Inaccurate measurement or recording is a particular concern when information comes from secondary data sources that are not designed for research or epidemiologic surveillance of medical care. For instance, Jollis *et al*[7] compared information about cardiac risk factors in an administrative database in patients undergoing angiography with information collected prospectively for a clinical database. A chance-corrected measure of agreement (kappa statistic) showed moderate to poor agreement as follows: hypertension (56%), heart failure (39%), and unstable angina (9%). Hannan *et al*[8] found similar discrepancies in comparing a cardiac surgery registry to an administrative database in New York State. While the accuracy of coding in administrative databases appears to be improving over time,[9,10] significant undercoding of comorbidities still exists, especially among the elderly.[10,11]

As noted above, limited or inaccurate data in insurance databases or computerized hospital discharge abstracts may be supplemented or corrected by chart audits. A more efficient approach is to establish registries geared to measuring key patient characteristics, process-of-care elements, and relevant outcomes. Registries are proliferating in cardiovascular medicine and surgery, especially for acute ischemic syndromes and coronary surgery. This has led, however, to a new challenge – that is, agreement on a set of core data elements and definitions so that reliable comparisons can be drawn across registries from different jurisdictions.

Key measures

Processes of care

Process of care is an umbrella term, encompassing all inputs into the clinical encounter that are relevant to the effectiveness and efficiency of the service provided. Process measures of particular interest for this chapter are the clinical decision-making patterns of physicians and other health professionals, as these reflect the uptake and use of evidence from the literature of medicine. Other inputs may also be relevant, such as hospital staffing ratios and qualifications of providers. Not infrequently, researchers use characteristics of the admitting hospital as ecologic proxies for processes of care that may affect individual patients.[12–14] In this respect, hospital volumes for specific diagnoses or procedures are often taken as proxies for the expertise or experience of the relevant providers. Some measures are intermediate. Waiting times for services and lengths of stay, for example, are at once indicators of the process of care, and outcomes of interest to patients, professionals, and administrators alike.

Outcomes

The most important outcomes studies in cardiovascular care are conventional randomized trials used to test the efficacy of novel interventions, as described elsewhere in this volume. However, non-randomized outcomes studies have a role in assessing practice patterns. These studies allow for the evaluation of therapies and the natural history of disease in real-world settings.[15,16] In some cases where randomization is simply not feasible (for example, socioeconomic status as a factor in prognosis), they also allow us to isolate patient characteristics from process-of-care factors to help elucidate pathophysiologic mechanisms of disease.[17,18] Perhaps most importantly, a cardiovascular service may be provided to the right patient at the right time, and for the right reasons, but be delivered in a technically substandard fashion that leads to needlessly poor outcomes. Non-randomized outcomes studies are therefore useful indicators of quality of care for technically demanding services.[19]

Outcomes of interest, after Kerr White, can be conveniently remembered as the six "Ds": death, disease, dysfunction, disability, distress, and dissatisfaction.[20] The easiest outcomes for health services researchers to measure are those that are defined objectively and usually captured in large insurance databases or computerized hospital administrative data. These include death, routinely-coded complications following surgery, or hospital re-admissions. Linkage to vital status registries is also performed to track out-of-hospital deaths. Unfortunately, health services researchers have often failed to assess other outcomes, such as functional status, symptom relief, or overall quality of life, that are very important to patients and their physicians.[21]

Assessing processes and outcomes of care

Assessing processes of care

Descriptive studies

Health services research gained considerable momentum in the 1970s and 1980s from studies pioneered by Wennberg and Gittelsohn,[22,23] which documented unexplained geographic variations in rates of services. These early studies were a population-wide extension of research done in single hospitals or in public and private prepayment plans starting in the 1930s and showed variations in how different physicians managed apparently similar patients. However, Wennberg and coworkers coupled computerized systems of hospital discharge abstracts to census data and showed that citizens living in one area were significantly more or less likely to undergo certain procedures than those living in other areas. They also showed that greater variations were generally demonstrable when procedures were more discretionary or elective, or where there was uncertainty about the indications for the procedure or service of interest.[24,25] In these latter instances, values and circumstances apparently interact strongly with evidence in driving decisions about service provision.[26]

Such descriptive studies continue to appear in the health services literature. They involve simple rates or proportions, with various numerators and denominators. Possible numerators include primary care visits or encounters, specialized diagnostic and therapeutic services, composite measures of use, such as overall numbers of hospital bed-days used per 10 000 residents, or even mean expenditures per capita on health care for all types of services. Denominators may tally patients according to the clinics or hospitals that they use, or by their residency in a given geographic area. These two denominators may be melded into hospital market shares – for example, the total population living in an area where a specified percentage of all patients receive their cardiac care at the hospital of interest.

Several statistical summary measures are used in variations analyses.[27,28] Computational details and statistical properties of these measures are beyond the scope of this chapter. What matters is that the degree of variation should be both statistically significant and suggestive of meaningful differences from the standpoint of quality, accessibility, or efficiency of care provision. Thus, examination of the patterns of service and potential outcome implications is arguably more illuminating than the focusing on specific summary measures.

The interpretive challenges of such descriptive studies are illustrated by evidence assembled with clinical and/or administrative data showing sex differences in treatments for patients hospitalized with acute myocardial infarction (AMI).[29–31] Sex differences in care have been found in several nations, but the relationship between gender and service intensity is not consistent.[32–34] The debate about the gender gap in service intensity is likely to continue until there is clearer evidence from randomized trials to delineate whether and how men and women with otherwise similar cardiovascular disease should be managed differently.

Variations in processes of care have been well documented to extend beyond patient factors. As one example of this genre, Chen *et al*[35] documented significant interhospital variations in length of stay after AMI in Ontario. These variations persisted after adjustment for various factors such as coronary angiography on the index admission, patients' age and sex, and comorbidity as inferred from secondary diagnoses on discharge abstracts. In almost any jurisdiction and for almost any cardiovascular service where interpractitioner, interinstitutional, or interregional variations in patterns of service provision have been sought, they are demonstrable.

In sum, descriptive studies showing process-of-care variations are tantamount to screening tests in medical practice. They raise the possibility that there may be a problem with quality, efficiency, or accessibility. However, the finding of statistically significant variations is predicated on a null hypothesis that processes of care should vary no more than would be expected on the basis of the play of chance. Most such studies apply direct or indirect standardization to control for differences in the age–sex profile of the populations being compared, but may not consider myriad other sources of variation (Box 8.1). In response to that limitation, researchers may either develop evidence-oriented criteria to examine decision making at the level of the individual case, or try to link processes and outcomes of care in the same study as a means of inferring a causal connection. We examine both types of studies below.

Box 8.1 Sources of regional/institutional variation in service profiles

- Age and sex composition
- Age/sex specific disease incidence
- Random variation with time and place
- Availability and practice organization, such as
  - primary care
  - specialist services
  - hospital services/bed provision
  - overall funding levels
  - methods of payment
  - alternative services
- Referral patterns
- Practice styles of service providers
- Variations in patient expectations, demands, health education/behaviors
- Rates of previous service (for example, organ removal where relevant)

Criteria-based utilization analyses

Given the limitations of descriptive studies that delineate variations in processes of care, health services researchers have developed other methods to determine whether the right service is provided to the right type of patient for the right reasons at the right time and place. One approach is implicit reviews of case records, drawing on the individualized judgments of expert clinicians. Unfortunately, lack of standardization renders implicit reviews unreliable.[36,37] Explicit criteria, which form the basis for most process-of-care analyses in the literature, have the advantages of standardization and consistency, as well as transparency. Where necessary, trained staff can apply them retrospectively to medical records without a major time commitment from clinicians. These studies are described in America as "utilization reviews" and in the UK as "clinical audits".[38]

Process-of-care audits have the advantage of efficiency in comparison to outcomes studies as quality management tools. Bad outcomes caused by negligence and incompetence are (happily) rare. Technical competence does not necessarily equate with good judgment and appropriateness of service provision. Moreover, bad outcomes from *under*-treatment are hard to detect because the impact of modern cardiovascular care is often to make life only a little better on average for patients or to reduce their risk of otherwise rare events. For example, from overviews of randomized placebo-controlled trials we know that β blockers confer about a 25% *relative* reduction in mortality in the first year after a myocardial infarction. For a cohort of medium-risk patients, this equates to an *absolute* reduction in cumulative postdischarge mortality from 4% to 3%. To show such a mortality difference on a comparative outcomes audit of two practices (80% power, 2-sided alpha of 0·05), we require over 5000 patients per practice; but a 1% mortality difference presumes absolutely no use of β blockers in the practice with poorer outcomes. A more realistic assumption would be that about 70% of eligible patients receive β blockers in the practice with worse outcomes versus over 95%

in the exemplary practice. Based on the randomized trials, this equates to perhaps a 0·2% increase in mortality. To detect such a small difference in mortality would require over 100 000 patients per practice! In contrast, one could simply examine charts to see whether patients were getting β blocker prescriptions, versus 70% in the other practice, one would only need to examine about 75 charts in each practice for a reliable assessment.

This latter audit is simple in another respect. We can basically use randomized trial inclusion and exclusion criteria to decide who should be getting the drug, make sure there are no obvious contraindications or medication intolerances documented on the medical record, and tally whether patients are getting the treatment that they ought to be getting. In general, however, audits require close attention to the validity, application, and applicability of the criteria chosen (Box 8.2).[38]

Box 8.2 User's guide to appraising and applying the results of a process-of-care audit

- *Are the criteria valid?*
  - Was an explicit and sensible process used to identify, select, and combine evidence for the criteria?
  - What is the quality of the evidence used in framing the criteria?
  - If necessary, was an explicit, systematic, and reliable process used to tap expert opinion?
  - Was an explicit and sensible process used to consider the relative values of different outcomes?
  - If the quality of the evidence used in originally framing the criteria was weak, have the criteria themselves been correlated with patient outcomes?
- *Were the criteria applied appropriately?*
  - Was the process of applying the criteria reliable, unbiased, and likely to yield robust conclusions?
  - What is the impact of uncertainty associated with evidence and values on the criteria-based ratings of process of care?
- *Can you use the criteria in your own practice setting?*
  - Are the criteria relevant to your practice setting?
  - Have the criteria been field-tested for feasibility of use in diverse settings, including settings similar to yours?

Adapted from Naylor and Guyatt[38]

Validity of audit criteria

To be valid, the criteria must have a direct link either to improving health (as is obvious with β blockers for secondary prevention after AMI) or to lowering resource use without compromising health outcomes. There should be an explicit and sensible process to identify, select, and combine the relevant outcomes-based evidence.

The hierarchy of evidence outlined above by Kitching, Sackett and Yusuf applies here. Evidence from randomized trials is strongly preferred, but evidence from observational sources cannot be ignored. For example, from observational studies within trials, it is plain that the largest survival benefits with thrombolytic therapy are obtained when treatment is administered early.[39] It would be unethical to randomize patients to receive thrombolysis on a delayed or urgent basis to determine how large these effects are. Thus, guidelines now recommend that thrombolytic therapy be administered, wherever possible, within 30 minutes of a pateint's arrival to hospital.[40] Studies from America,[41] Canada,[42] the UK,[43] Italy,[44] and New Zealand[45] have all documented remediable problems with treatment delays in administering thrombolytic agents to eligible patients. All are classic examples of criteria-based audits.

If only some of the indications for a particular service under audit will be covered by high quality evidence, then weaker sources of evidence, inference, and expert opinion must often be brought into play, usually through formal panel processes. Such panels should include an explicit process for selecting panelists, and a sensible, systematic method for collating their judgments. In this respect, the RAND group has pioneered multispecialty panel methods that are widely emulated.[46–48] Scenarios are compiled that describe a potential indication for the procedure or clinical service in question. Each expert panelist independently rates hundreds of different case scenarios on a risk–benefit scale. Scenarios are re-rated at a panel meeting after patterns of interpanelist agreement and disagreement are shown anonymously and discussed. The final set of panelists' ratings then determines whether a given indication is deemed potentially appropriate, uncertain, or inappropriate.

With this method, it is not clear whether the appropriateness ratings for any given indication rest primarily on research evidence or inference, extrapolation, and opinion. The relative values placed on different outcomes are also unclear. For example, in randomized trials of CABG versus percutaneous transluminal coronary angioplasty (PTCA),[49–52] PTCA has a slightly lower early mortality, along with lower initial costs and more rapid recovery from the procedure. Longer term mortality data are similar, but CABG patients appear to achieve better symptom relief, have decreased use of medication, and require fewer subsequent procedures.[53] When an expert panel addresses the respective appropriateness of PTCA and CABG, the findings reflect these trade offs, but we cannot be sure that patients themselves would make the same choices. The conflation of facts and values in panel-based criteria is highlighted by studies showing that the nationality of a panel markedly affects the criteria and results of applying them to cardiovascular procedures (Table 8.1).[26,54] Indeed, available evidence would also suggest that hospital practice settings and resource availability influence panel-based criteria.[55] Nonetheless, the RAND methods compare very favorably with those used to create several utilization review tools now in widespread use.[38]

Table 8.1 Categorization of appropriateness of indications for cardiovascular procedures based on actual audits in the field: cross-national differences in expert panel assessments

Procedure	Location/sample	Year	*n*	Panel nationality	Appropriate	Uncertain	Inappropriate
Coronary artery bypass graft	USA, 4 hospitals in Washington State	1979–80	386	American	62	25	13
		1979–82		British	41	24	35
	UK, 3 hospitals in Trent region	1987–88	319	American	67	26	7
				British	57	27	16
	Canada, 13 hospitals in Ontario and British Columbia	1989–90	556	American	88	9	3
				Canadian	85	11	4
	USA, 15 hospitals in New York State	1990	1336	American	91	7	2
				Canadian	85	10	6
Coronary angiography	USA, 4 hospitals in Washington State	1979–80	376	American	50	23	27
		1979–82		British	11	29	60
	USA, Medicare beneficiaries in 3 states	1981	1677	American	74	9	17
				British	39	19	42
	UK, 3 hospitals in Trent region	1987–88	320	American	71	12	17
				British	49	30	21
	Canada, 20 hospitals in Ontario and British Columbia	1989–90	533	American	77	18	5
				Canadian	58	33	9
	USA, 15 hospitals in New York State	1990	1333	American	76	20	4
				Canadian	51	39	10

Adapted from Naylor[26]
The data show the appropriateness ratings for sets of identical patient charts as described. Each set of charts was assessed according to criteria derived by expert panels based in the listed countries.

Application and applicability of the audit criteria

Application of explicit process-of-care criteria often rests on data derived from retrospective chart reviews by professional auditors. The audit process must therefore be reliable. Biases can be introduced through skewed sampling of practitioners, hospitals, and patients. Even a meticulous audit, however, may miss mitigating factors. Thus, in many instances, if the explicit review shows potential problems with the appropriateness of a service, the case is assessed by experienced clinicians to preclude "false positives".

It is also crucial that enough cases be reviewed to draw robust conclusions. For example, in one study, RAND researchers used explicit criteria to assess the appropriateness of PTCA in 1990 for 1306 randomly selected patients in 15 randomly selected New York State hospitals.[54] The inappropriate utilization rate varied by hospital from 1% to

9% ($P = 0{\cdot}12$). Differences of this magnitude, if real, could be important to patients, payers, and policy makers. Thus, this sample size may have been insufficient for the investigators to confirm important differences in quality among hospitals.

Although the task is subjective, end users must consider intangibles such as local medical culture and practice circumstances before accepting audit criteria that may not be relevant. The stronger the evidence on which the criteria are based, the less one needs to consider local factors; for example, few medical cultures would reject aspirin for AMI – a cheap and simple drug treatment that has been definitively proven to yield reductions in mortality. With weaker evidence and higher costs, however, the judgments are less straightforward.

Last, even if criteria are sufficiently valid and relevant, training times and other costs must be considered. Special logistical problems arise when criteria are used for concurrent case management rather than retrospective utilization review. Any errors associated with concurrent care management will have immediate consequences for individual patients and physicians. Nonetheless, many American hospitals already do a range of concurrent reviews.

The use of chart audits to infer appropriateness

Table 8.1 shows the proportion of appropriate, inappropriate, and "uncertain" indications for cardiac procedures as randomly audited in the USA, UK, and Canada.[26,56–58] Since all the procedures shown are used many times more often in the USA than in the UK, it seems almost paradoxical that the proportions of inappropriate cases are not much higher in the USA. The literature has suggested that relationships between appropriateness of care and cardiovascular service intensity are similarly weak within nations.[25,58–60]

However, two studies shed a slightly different light on this issue. The rates of all major coronary procedures in New York State, USA are about twice as high as in Ontario, Canada.[61] Figure 8.1 shows the relative rate of isolated coronary artery bypass surgery (CABG) for the two jurisdictions by age and anatomy. Overall, only 6% of CABG patients in Ontario versus 30% of patients in New York had limited coronary artery disease – one or two vessel disease without proximal left anterior descending (PLAD) involvement. However, more patients in New York had left mainstem disease (23% *v* 16%, $P < 0{\cdot}001$). In relative terms, the differences are most dramatic among elderly persons. For example, New York brings 17 times as many persons over the age of 75 to surgery with anatomic patterns of coronary disease that are not associated with life expectancy gains after CABG. Nonetheless, much of this extra use could pass an appropriateness audit, since 90% of the persons with limited coronary anatomic disease in New York had moderate to severe angina before surgery.[61]

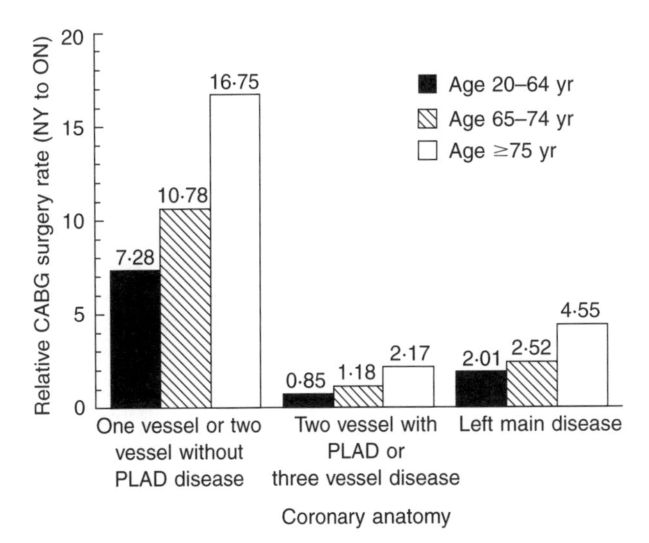

Figure 8.1 Relative rate of isolated CABG for New York State (NY) and Ontario (ON) according to age and disease anatomy. Adapted from Tu *et al*.[61] PLAD, proximal left anterior descending.

A reasonable inference is that major increases in capacity, and expansion of population-based services rates, are associated with *diminishing marginal returns*. The Canadian approach – fixed budgets in a universal health system, and "managed delay" with organized waiting lists[62] – seems to promote more efficient use of resources, with patients receiving surgery primarily if they are likely to have life expectancy gain. However, restricted use of coronary angiography leads to some implicit rationing that affects primarily the elderly, and a certain proportion of patients at all ages with left mainstem disease are not detected and/or do not undergo surgery.

A second study[63] of CABG develops this argument more strongly. Rather than using appropriateness criteria from an expert panel, Hux *et al* based their case-specific process assessments on a meta-analysis of randomized trials by Yusuf *et al*[64] Whereas the broad category of "appropriate" care as defined by expert panels includes a range of risk–benefit ratios, a trials-based assessment allowed estimation of the degree of potential 10 year survival benefit conferred by CABG surgery among patients for whom, by and large, it was appropriate. Hux *et al* found that only 6% of 5058 Ontario patients undergoing isolated CABG in 1992–93 fell in the low benefit category – that is, patients for whom there is no survival advantage from early CABG. However, the degree of anticipated benefit differed according to the center where surgery was provided. For instance, the proportion of patients in a high-benefit category ranged from 65·2 to 79·9% ($P < 0{\cdot}001$). Significantly more patients were in a high-benefit category in hospitals serving areas with lower population-based rates of CABG. Analyzing the data by site of residence, there was an inverse relationship between marginal degree of life expectancy gains and the surgical rates for each county.[63]

In sum, if one accepts that overtly inappropriate services are unlikely to be commonplace in any health system, the relationship between appropriateness of care and population-based services rates can be redefined. Rather than seeking to relate the prevalence of bad judgment to high service intensity, or decrying health systems with low service intensity for rationing care, researchers might better assess whether the marginal returns of other forms of cardiovascular care are indeed smaller in areas where those services are used more frequently. The policy decision then becomes one of trade offs: given competing demands on scarce healthcare resources, at what point do the marginal returns of particular cardiac services become low enough that further investment in those services cannot be justified?

Evidence-oriented clinicians must be positioned to contribute to these debates by marshaling comparative utilization data that help decision makers make explicit determination of the likely yields from funding different sets of cardiovascular and non-cardiovascular services. Arguably, they must also use these evaluative tools to safeguard their patients against inappropriate *underuse* of necessary services.

Again, explicit process-of-care criteria can be helpful. For example, analytical variations studies using American data have repeatedly shown that black and uninsured patients have lower coronary angiography rates than those who are insured.[65–67] Laouri *et al*[68] drew on audit data from four teaching hospitals in Los Angeles and assembled a cohort of 352 patients who met explicitly defined criteria for the necessity of coronary angiography as established by an expert panel. The patients were tracked forward for 3 months and, after adjustment for confounding factors, those managed in the public hospital system had a 35% rate of angiography versus 57% for private hospital patients ($P<0{\cdot}005$).

Two recent studies incorporate appropriateness criteria to provide further evidence for underuse of coronary interventions. The first by Guadagnoli *et al*[69] examined variations in coronary angiography after AMI in approximately 50 000 elderly Medicare beneficiaries in the USA. Among those patients with ACC–AHA class 1 indications, coronary angiography was used less often among Medicare beneficiaries enrolled in managed-care plans than among those with fee-for-service coverage. Moreover, utilization rates among elderly patients with class I indications for angiography were low in both groups (37% *v* 46%), suggesting room for improving the care of such patients with acute myocardial infarction. In contrast, the rate of angiography use among those with ACC–AHA class III indications (where angiography was deemed not useful) was similarly low (13%) in both groups. The second prospective study applied appropriateness ratings for coronary revascularization procedures to 2552 patients identified at the time of coronary angiography for various indications. Among 908 patients with indications appropriate for PTCA, 34% were treated medically. Among 1353 patients with indications appropriate for CABG, 26% were treated medically. Relating processes to outcomes, the research team also found that medically-treated patients deemed appropriate for revascularization were more likely to experience adverse events downstream.[70]

The lesson, simply put, is that evidence must be sought for both inappropriate *overuse* and *underuse* of cardiovascular services in any and all healthcare systems.

Outcomes studies and process–outcome relationships

Types of outcome studies

Researchers, clinicians, and administrators alike are also drawing on outcomes with increasing frequency as a means of assessing quality of care. To repeat a point made earlier, various biases threaten the validity of inferences drawn from these non-randomized studies; but they have a useful role both in monitoring quality of care and as a source of evidence when randomization is not feasible or appropriate.

Just as studies in the 1960s and 1970s showed geographic and institutional variations in broad markers of processes of care, so also did the 1980s and 1990s see the publication of research demonstrating significant mortality differences across physicians,[71] hospitals,[72] regions,[73] and health systems.[74] The magnitude of mortality variations has been meaningful, even amongst relatively homogeneous groups of patients. For example, Tu *et al* demonstrated marked interhospital and interregional variations in 1 year risk-adjusted mortality rates for patients hospitalized between 1994 and 1997 in one Canadian province. Mortality ranged from 20·8% to 27·4% across regions, and from 17·6% to 32·3% across hospitals admitting 100 or more AMI cases per year.[75] Regional variations persist even in highly selected subpopulations of patients. Pilote *et al* demonstrated that 1 year AMI mortality rate across eight US census regions ranged from 8·6% to 10·3% among the population enrolled in GUSTO-1.[73]

As with descriptive studies of variations in process of care, these high-level outcomes studies function largely as screening tests: they often raise more questions than answers. Researchers use multivariate analyses to adjust for prognostic differences in the patient populations being compared. However, since patients are not randomized to different sites or regions, there is uncertainty about the extent to which unmeasured variation in patient characteristics accounts for the residual outcomes variation. Furthermore, the higher the level of comparison and the longer the follow up, the more uncertain the causal inferences become. Regional differences in long-term AMI outcomes, for example, may reflect genetic differences in populations, environmental factors, regional variation in health behaviors and socioeconomic status, as well as more conventional factors such as variations in processes of care on the index hospitalization and follow up interventions (for example, revascularization or rehabilitation).

For convenience, we suggest that outcomes analyses in health services research can be classified variously as *quality-of-care screening studies* or *process/outcome hypothesis studies.*

Quality-of-care screening studies focus on outcomes to detect variations in quality of care. They are most powerful when applied to short-term outcomes that are closely tied to a particular episode of illness or procedure, and a provider or institution. In these circumstances, causal inferences are more straightforward. Their applicability is clearest for technically demanding procedures, such as PTCA or CABG, where variations in outcomes are taken as proxies for operator skill. However, even in such instances, other factors in pre- and perioperative care may be important. For relatively homogeneous diagnoses, outcomes studies may also sometimes be a useful screen to determine if detailed process-of-care analyses are required. For example, if inhospital mortality were found to be similarly low across a whole set of institutions, there would be little rationale for undertaking a major audit of processes of care.

Ultimately, the goal of such studies is to isolate one or more process-of-care factors that can be modified to lead to consistently better outcomes. Outcomes analyses may also be used to validate process-of-care criteria or their application, for example, the study of underuse of revascularization by Hemingway *et al* cited above.[70] In this sense there is overlap between the two categories of non-randomized outcomes studies. But an important distinction should also be drawn. Quality-of-care studies are concerned with the applicability of existing evidence in a particular context. Other outcomes studies may be initiated with a view to deriving or supporting generalizable hypotheses about the process–outcome relationship. They are poor cousins to randomized trials from the standpoint of strength of evidence. For true efficacy assessments, randomized trials are usually possible and always preferable, given the unavoidable biases of observational studies.[76] A poorly conducted non-randomized outcomes comparison for quality management purposes may at worst mislead patients and tarnish the reputation of a number of capable cardiologists or cardiac surgeons. A poorly conducted non-randomized outcome comparison of two treatments may, if taken seriously, misguide clinical practice worldwide.

That caveat aside, these process/outcome hypothesis studies can be useful to illustrate unanticipated harm from interventions, test the external validity of randomized trial results, generate hypotheses about interventions that may be worth testing with formal experimental designs, and, in special circumstances, provide an acceptable level of evidence for adopting a particular intervention.

There are many methods available for examining the relationship between processes of care and outcomes. The simplest method is to draw broad causal inferences using ecological comparisons, for example, correlating differences in processes and outcomes across two or more institutions or jurisdictions. However, the greater the difference between service settings being compared, the more difficult it is to be sure that patients were similar, or to isolate which aspects, if any, of the process of care relate to the outcomes observed. This is especially true when comparisons are made on a broad geographic footing between regions or countries in which populations and processes of care differ in many ways. In these latter comparisons, we are obviously veering away from the use of non-randomized outcomes data to benchmark technical quality of care for homogeneous procedures, and entering the more complex realm of process/outcome hypothesis studies.

This genre is typified by several studies[77–80] showing that Canadian patients have more symptoms, worse functional status, or higher death/re-admission rates after AMI than do American patients. The reasons for these differences, however, are unclear. For example, Mark *et al*[78] in a GUSTO-1 substudy found that, while rates of revascularization were much higher in the USA, Canadians drew their post-MI care more often from family physicians and general internists, while Americans relied more on cardiologists and received more cardiac rehabilitation services.[78] In other words, revascularization was only one factor among many that might explain differences in outcomes across two health systems.

In an effort to limit the effects of competing process factors, analysts have borrowed the concept of instrumental variables from econometrics.[81] This approach compares patients' outcomes according to some characteristic that sharply distinguishes the care of two or more groups of patients. Thus, one might attempt to elucidate the impact of differences in the rate of revascularization across hospitals with and without on-site interventional capacity. Alter *et al*[72] recently used such a design to show that hospitals with on-site revascularization facilities had a lower rate of non-fatal composite outcomes (recurrent cardiac hospitalization and emergency department visits), and were also 3·5 times more likely to refer patients to myocardial revascularization procedures. Yet, despite the markedly higher rates of invasive procedures, the non-fatal outcome advantages of invasive-procedure hospitals were actually explained by their teaching status!

In sum, given the relatively weak inferences possible from most observational studies of outcomes, alternative strategies for ensuring the quality of medical care should always be considered. It will often be feasible and more efficient to use randomized trials or meta-analyses of trials to establish optimal management strategies, and then ensure that quality of care is maintained by monitoring the process of care in that well-proven practices are consistently applied to eligible patients. On the other hand, for high volume and technically demanding procedures where reasonable risk adjustment methods can be brought into play, outcomes measurement has merit for quality control so long as the results are interpreted carefully. Finally, studies aimed at delineating process–outcome relationships will continue to be valuable, but researchers and evidence-oriented practitioners alike will often find that the interpretation of the findings plunges them into a thicket of causes, effects, and epiphenomena.

Special challenges in non-randomized outcomes studies

In this section, we delve more deeply into some of the analytical challenges of non-randomized outcomes studies. Many types of biases have been described in the literature,[82,83] but selection bias is a recurrent concern whether one is comparing the outcomes of two cardiac surgeons, or using non-randomized data to develop hypotheses about the effectiveness of pharmacologic or non-pharmacologic therapies in real-world settings. Indeed, the ubiquity of selection bias in health services research arises from the fact that ordinary good judgment in practice inevitably means that there are systematic differences in the characteristics of patients who are selected for particular interventions as compared to those who are not.

Patients selected post-MI to undergo coronary angiography, for example, are often younger and healthier than other MI victims.[72,82] The survival benefits observed for those undergoing angiography may therefore be due to prognostic characteristics rather than to revascularization consequent upon angiography. This latter phenomenon is known as confounding and is a common result of selection biases. Confounding occurs when particular factors are associated with both a study (process) variable and the outcome of interest.

Researchers therefore routinely employ some form of multivariate analysis to adjust for imbalances in prognostic factors between groups under study. A complementary strategy is to confirm the consistency of the findings after restricting the analysis to a relatively *low*-risk subgroup of the patients being examined.[76] Eliminating patients in higher risk categories associated with more widely varying physiologic states increases the likelihood of a "level playing field" for comparisons.

For many common procedures and diagnoses, researchers can draw on validated prognostic indices and risk-adjustment algorithms as signposts in carrying out study-specific multivariate analyses. For frequently studied procedures such as CABG, major studies have tended to show relative consistency in the types of prognostic clinical factors that must be taken into account for risk adjustment purposes.[84] Not surprisingly, risk-adjustment models appear to perform somewhat better with clinical as compared to administrative data.[85] However, the key to predictive performance appears to be better data, not more variables. Studies have suggested that the accuracy of risk-adjustment models reaches a plateau after use of only a few key variables. Tu *et al*,[86] for example, examined risk-adjusted hospital mortality rates for CABG with multisite registry data. They determined that six core variables in a risk-adjustment model (age, gender, emergency surgery, previous CABG, LV dysfunction, left main disease) permitted modest discrimination between patients who did and did not die postoperatively (area under the receiver operating characteristic [ROC] curve = 0·77). Statistical performance improved only trivially with the inclusion of six additional characteristics, and the relative rankings in the risk-adjusted mortality rates between hospitals did not change. Notwithstanding these studies, the ultimate number as well as the type of clinical variables required in a risk-adjustment model will obviously depend upon the disease being assessed, the processes and outcomes of interest, and the unit of analysis (for example, risk-adjusted mortality rates per physician *v* per hospital).

Propensity scores can also be used to contain the impact of confounding.[87] This method reduces the entire collection of background characteristics into a single composite characteristic (that is, the propensity to receive treatment *v* no treatment), which is then used to subclassify patients further into categories of relative equal propensities. Accordingly, the case-mix composition of patients with similar propensities is balanced, and outcome differences can be directly compared between those receiving and not receiving treatment.

While not a solution for confounding *per se*, hierarchical statistical modeling has recently found favor as a useful analytical tool in outcome studies.[88,89] Data in health research frequently exist in an ordered hierarchical structure: that is, patients are managed by physicians who practice within hospitals. In contrast, traditional multivariate techniques ignore the natural hierarchy of data and treat each observation as if it were independent (Figure 8.2).

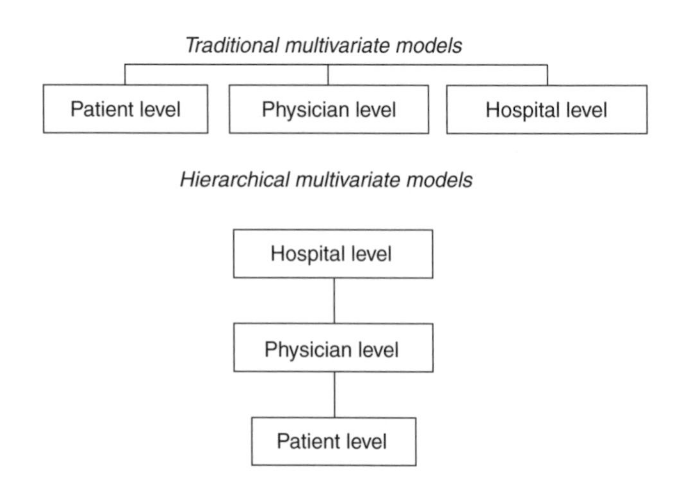

Figure 8.2 Schematic view of hierarchical *v* traditional models

The use of hierarchical modeling makes intuitive sense since patients may share higher-level characteristics, leading to observations that are not necessarily independent of one another. The existence of standardized inhospital processes of care (for example, treatment protocols and care maps) may result in greater homogeneity in treatments across patients admitted to a particular institution. Accordingly, the use of traditional multivariate analyses may lead to an artificially inflated number of independent observations and an underestimate in the magnitude of standard error and potential alpha error.[90]

While the embedding of multivariate analyses in a hierarchical structure has obvious advantages, neither this technique nor fastidious risk-adjustment methods can match the effectiveness of randomization when balancing the case-mix distribution between two groups, especially because researchers and quality-of-care evaluators are unlikely to know all the prognostic factors that interact with processes of care and may alter outcomes. Moreover, even if key prognostic confounders are known, they may not all have been measured or recorded accurately. Box 8.3 sets out some general principles that may be useful when researchers appraise non-randomized outcome studies.[38]

Box 8.3 User's guide to appraising an observational outcomes study

- Are the outcome measures accurate and comprehensive?
- Were there clearly identified, sensible comparison groups?
- Were all important determinants of outcome measured accurately and reliably?
- Were the comparison groups similar with respect to important determinants, other than the one of interest?
- Was multivariate analysis used to adjust for imbalances in patient prognostic factors and other outcome determinants?
- Did additional analyses (particularly in low-risk subgroups) demonstrate the same results as the primary analysis?
- Did any multivariate analysis take into account natural heirarchies in the data, such as clustering of patients within providers' practices and/or within institutions?

Adapted from Naylor and Guyatt[38]

Changing practice patterns

General considerations

Practices clearly change over time in response to published evidence. At times, these changes can be rapid and dramatic, particularly when an innovation is associated with overwhelmingly positive risk–benefit ratios and is feasible for large numbers of practitioners to adopt. This model of knowledge-based practice change is termed *passive diffusion*. Its impact is heightened by the extent to which the mass media pick up major medical advances, and by the marketing initiatives of drug and device manufacturers. However, as implied by studies showing unexplained and undesirable variations in practice patterns, the model of passive diffusion leads to inconsistent uptake of evidence into practice.

How, then, can evidence be incorporated into practice more consistently, and what happens when data are in hand showing either that practice departs sharply from what available evidence suggests should be the norm, or that technical competence is below standard? How can the gap between "is" and "ought" in medical care be closed? These questions relate to changing physician (and system) performance, and follow logically from work done to measure or assess practice processes and outcomes.

Although there is limited randomized evidence on this topic for specific aspects of cardiovascular care, a wealth of experience – some unhappy – has shown that direct incentives and disincentives, financial and otherwise, can have a major impact on practice. Bonuses are paid in American managed care organizations if practitioners meet certain financial and clinical performance targets. Within the UK National Health Service, meeting targets for prespecified preventive services leads to extra payments for general practitioners; and the new rating system for hospital trusts offers administrative autonomy and preferential access to capital funding as a reward for strong performance on measures of quality, accessibility, and efficiency. Simply shifting the mode of physician payment may be an effective way of modifying behavior. For example, exponents of fee-for-service remuneration of cardiovascular medicine and surgery argue that salary and capitation schemes impose a risk of underservicing. Critics of fee-for-service argue that it undervalues quality and cognitive services, and creates a conflict of interest that promotes the use of procedures. As to non-financial incentives and disincentives, the range of options includes merit awards, disciplinary proceedings, and litigation.

Arguably more relevant to the evidence-oriented practitioner is the available information on non-administrative mechanisms to improve physician performance that rely on voluntary knowledge- or information-based change. Such initiatives have the advantage of calling forward the better instincts of health professionals who, with few exceptions, seek first to serve patients as competently as possible.

Exponents of clinical guidelines initially believed that dissemination of guidelines might prove a key component in catalyzing knowledge-based improvements in physician performance.[91] Guidelines would usefully compile the totality of relevant evidence on several related aspects of a clinical condition, treatment, or procedure. The evidence-oriented practitioner would no longer have to comb through the clinical literature, critically appraise it, and keep the relevant materials at hand or in her/his memory. The guideline would instead provide a convenient source of definitive evidence. Furthermore, because inference, expert judgment, values, and circumstances could be used in developing guidelines, clinicians would be able to rely on regionally-developed guidelines to navigate the many "grey zones" of clinical practice[26] where evidence alone was insufficient. Finally, guidelines could be developed, endorsed and disseminated by authorities with clinical credibility, lending weight to evidence that might otherwise appear rather impersonally in clinical journals.

Lomas[92] termed this latter approach the model of *active dissemination*, and criticized its prospects for success on the grounds that it ignored other factors in the practice environment, and presupposed that information acquisition alone leads to behavior change. The available evidence does suggest that there is some impact from more active approaches to informing and educating physicians about relevant clinical advances or guideline content.[93] However, the more passive the educational process, and the more removed it is from physicians' own practice context, the less likely it appears to succeed.

Researchers and administrators have accordingly developed an array of non-coercive interventions designed to improve physician performance (Box 8.4). In 1995 Davis *et al*[94] and Oxman *et al*[95] conducted systematic reviews of all the available controlled studies of the effects of these strategies on physicians' and other health professionals' performance. They included any strategy designed to persuade physicians "to modify their practice performance by communicating clinical information". Purely administrative interventions or financial and similar applied incentives and disincentives were excluded.

There were 99 studies involving physicians and a further three on other health professionals' behavior. Most of the studies on physician performance focus on internists or family physicians, and specific cardiovascular studies are limited in number to date. Single-intervention studies had positive effects on process or outcome parameters in 49/81 (60%) of trials where they were applied. Short educational seminars or conferences and dissemination of educational materials (printed or in audiovisual format) were least effective of all the single-intervention modalities explored. This finding supports proponents of implementation as opposed to dissemination.

Simple audit-and-feedback studies had limited impact. However, it is important to distinguish the types of studies that fall into this category. For example, in randomized studies from the early 1980s, investigators showed that a computer-based monitoring system with reminders and feedback led to significantly better follow up and blood pressure control for patients with hypertension.[96,97] Two controlled studies by Pozen *et al*[98,99] showed that a point-of-service strategy to facilitate implementation of a predictive algorithm for chest pain diagnosis reduced inappropriate use of coronary care units. These studies can best be regarded as "reminder" studies because there is continuous feedback at point of service. Audit-and-feedback studies that appear to be ineffective are those where data are collected and cumulated about processes or outcomes, and fed back only intermittently to practitioners without mechanisms to ensure local buy-in, to address local barriers to change, or to rectify specific gaps in clinical knowledge that may be associated with aberrant practice patterns.

The latter distinction also highlights the fact that feedback can occur concurrently with service provision or retrospectively (that is, after the service has been provided). Concurrent audit and feedback arguably is taken to its

Box 8.4 Some methods used to alter physician performance/behavior

- **Education materials:** Distribution of published or printed recommendations, including practice guidelines and audiovisual materials or electronic publications.
- **Conferences:** Participation of healthcare providers in conferences, lectures, workshops, or traineeships outside their practice settings.
- **Outreach visits:** Use of a trained person who meets with providers in their practice settings to provide information. The information given may include feedback on the provider's performance.
- **Local opinion leaders:** Use of providers explicitly nominated by their colleagues to be "educationally influential".
- **Patient-mediated interventions:** Any intervention aimed at changing the performance of healthcare providers for which information was sought from or given directly to patients by others (for example, direct mailings to patients, patient counseling delivered by others, or clinical information collected directly from patients and given to the provider).
- **Audit and feedback:** Any summary of clinical performance of healthcare over a specified period, with or without recommendations for clinical action. The information may have been obtained from medical records, computerized databases or patients or by observation.
- **Reminders:** Any intervention (manual or computerized) that prompts the healthcare provider to perform a clinical action. Examples include concurrent or intervisit reminders to professionals about desired actions such as screening or other preventive services, enhanced laboratory reports or administrative support (for example, follow up appointment systems or stickers on charts).
- **Marketing:** Use of personal interviewing, group discussion (focus groups) or a survey of targeted providers to identify barriers to change and the subsequent design of an intervention.
- **Local consensus processes:** Inclusion of participating providers in discussion to ensure agreement that the chosen clinical problem is important and the approach to managing it appropriate.

Modified from Oxman *et al*[95]

administrative conclusion in utilization management programs that refuse to authorize payment for a cardiovascular procedure unless the patient meets certain criteria, or in mandatory second opinion programs. These types of programs were not included in the reviews by Davis *et al*[94] and Oxman *et al.*[95]

The methods that had the most consistent effects were: outreach visits including formal academic detailing and opinion-leader studies, where an educationally influential physician was nominated by local peers to be the vector for the information; physician reminder systems at point of service; and patient-mediated methods, including reminders or educational materials. If two or more modalities were combined, then the effects were greater – that is, combining two effective methods (for example, academic detailing with support from a local opinion leader) had more impact than combining two less effective methods (for example, audit-and-feedback combined with a one-day seminar). Multifaceted interventions showed the strongest effects, with 31 of 39 (79%) positively affecting processes or outcomes of care.

Davis *et al*[94] noted that most interventions appear to have a greater impact on process-of-care measures and other indices of physician performance, than on patient outcomes. They postulated that this may be because the clinical interventions themselves have limited impact (a rationale for the power argument given earlier), and because patients do not always accept physician recommendations. They also suggest that a recurring weakness in interventions designed to improve processes and outcomes of care is a failure to conduct a needs analysis that addresses barriers to change.

These systematic reviews of practice-change interventions do not provide definitive evidence about which behavior change interventions are most effective and efficient in particular contexts or clinical conditions. This is because the studies cover a wide range of clinical condition and provider groups, rendering inferences across studies difficult. As in any meta-analysis, cross-study inferences involve non-randomized comparison with all their potential pitfalls. Furthermore, factorial designs in behavior changes studies have been more the exception than the rule, and it is therefore usually unclear as to which element(s) in a multifactorial strategy was (were) truly effective. Nonetheless, the evidence from controlled trials does suggest that practice changes are best achieved by combining credible evidence or information with active local strategies of implementation using multifactorial methods. Such multifactorial initiatives are further supported in a recent qualitative study examining factors leading to increasing β blocker use after AMI.[100] Hospitals with greater improvements in β blocker use over time, when compared to those having less or no improvement, were more likely to have shared goals, substantial administrative support, strong physician leadership advocating β blocker use, and incorporation of credible data feedback programs.

The case of outcomes report cards

The interest in outcomes measurement to assure technical competence has led to statewide initiatives whereby all cardiac surgery centers in New York and Pennsylvania, USA, are mandated to provide clinical data to permit compilation of publicly released mortality "report cards" on their CABG patients. (More recently, cardiovascular report cards have included interregional and hospital-specific AMI mortality rates, process indicators, (for example, evidence-based therapies and cardiac intervention rates post-AMI),[75,101] and patient satisfaction with hospital care.[102])

The CABG report cards provide a final case study that bridges some of the material presented above on outcomes assessment and behavior change. In New York between 1989 and 1992, inhospital postoperative mortality of CABG showed an unadjusted relative decline of 21%.[103,104] Patients were apparently becoming sicker in the same period, so that the risk-adjusted mortality decline was computed as 41%. Exponents of outcomes reporting claim that this improvement was catalyzed by a reporting system that provided relevant data to patients, administrators, and referring physicians.[103,104] There can be no doubt that the New York and Pennsylvania report cards have pinpointed problems with a few operators who had very poor technical outcomes. The key question is how much of the overall improvement in mortality can be attributed to public outcomes reportage.

Some critics contend that the trend is confounded by two factors. More assiduous coding of risk factors would artefactually increase the overall expected mortality, and surgeons could generate better mortality profiles by selectively turning down high-risk patients, even though such patients may have most to gain from CABG. There has indeed been a striking increase in the prevalence of various reported risk factors in the New York database since its inception. For example, prevalence of congestive heart failure rose from 1·7% in 1989 to 7·6% in 1991; renal failure rose from 0·4% to 2·8%, chronic obstructive pulmonary disease (COPD) from 6·9% to 17·4% and unstable angina from 14·9% to 21·8% in the same period.[105] As well, a survey[106] of randomly selected cardiologists and cardiac surgeons in Pennsylvania found that about 60% of cardiologists reported greater difficulty in finding surgeons who would operate on high-risk patients; a similar number of surgeons reported that they were less willing to operate on such patients. However, this type of survey is weak evidence for harm done by untoward case selection, and internal New York data do not support such a trend in the state.[107]

A more telling criticism is the fact that ecological correlations between falling mortality and initiation of reportage are tantamount to a case series in medicine. They provide weak and uncontrolled evidence for causation. In fact, the above-noted survey[106] of randomly selected cardiologists in Pennsylvania showed that most referring physicians did not view the Pennsylvania guide as an important source of information because of concerns about inadequate risk adjustment, unreliable data, and the absence of indicators of quality other than mortality. Schneider and Epstein[108] later surveyed patients undergoing cardiac surgery in Pennsylvania to determine the impact of the statewide consumer guide to the performance of hospitals and individual surgeons. Only 12% of the patients were aware of the guide before undergoing a CABG, and less than 1% knew the correct rating of their hospital or surgeon or reported that such information had any meaningful influence on their selection of a provider for open-heart surgery.

It is perhaps not surprising that, more generally, a recent overview by Marshall *et al*[109] found little evidence for consumer-driven market shifts arising from public report cards about specific diseases or procedures. It appears more plausible that the publication of outcomes "report cards" facilitates change by sensitizing politicians, public servants, and the governing bodies of hospitals to the existence of outcome variations. For example, after the publication of the CABG "report card", New York State insisted on attainment of center-specific minimum case volumes before certifying any cardiac surgery program.

On the other hand, in the absence of any report cards, the drop in post-CABG mortality in neighboring Massachusetts[110] has rivaled that seen in New York and Pennsylvania. Technical improvements in surgery, together with closer quality monitoring at the institutional level, appear to be the primary reason for these improved outcomes.

Given what has been learned about physician behavior change, the controversy about the New York State and Pennsylvania programs is hardly surprising. These externally mandated experiments in outcomes assessment contrast with initiatives that involve influential professionals and promote local buy-in from the outset. O'Connor discusses elsewhere in this volume the successful regional collaboration for continuous quality improvement that was developed in northern New England by involving cardiac surgeons in a systematic examination and improvement of processes and outcomes of care.[111–113] In Canada, a similar cooperative venture exists through the Cardiac Care Network of Ontario, which draws together representatives of all major cardiovascular referral centers in the province.[114] Historically, confidential report cards on mortality and length of stay were generated for the chief of cardiac surgery and CEO (cheif executive officer) at each center, using risk adjustment algorithms coauthored by leaders of the Cardiac Care Network itself.[84] CABG outcomes in Ontario are comparable to those in New York and Pennsylvania. Moreover, as in Massachusetts, the trend to improved outcomes antedates the report card system.[115,116] Most recently, hospital-specific CABG outcomes in Ontario have been made available to the public.

In summary, the unresolved issues with public outcomes report cards include validity and reliability of the data and the risk adjustment algorithms, as well as inadvertent adverse effects (for example, avoidance of high-risk patients, and consumers' or referring physicians' focus on point estimates rather than statistically reliable ranges). Potential harm to the public from substandard technical competence must be weighed against needless patient anxieties and confusion, along with harm to skilled health workers and fine institutions caused by poorly founded and widely publicized inferences about inferior outcomes. Debate continues, but it is untenable to assume that all hospitals or providers are equally technically competent, and the public has an unequivocal right to receive reliable and current data on physician and hospital performance. Thus, the trend must inexorably be toward greater public reporting of both process and outcome indicators of quality of care. The challenges for evidence-oriented practitioners are to ensure that the right indicators are chosen, that reliable data are analyzed appropriately, and that responsible reporting mechanisms are developed.

Conclusions

Assessing cardiovascular practices involves observational methods that can focus on either processes or outcomes of care. Methodologies for process-of-care assessments range from simple descriptive studies revealing variations in practice, to highly sophisticated case-specific audits using explicit criteria. Process-of-care assessments are more efficient than outcomes assessments in many respects, and lend themselves to measuring both over- and underuse of necessary cardiovascular services, thereby shedding light on quality and accessibility of care.

Observational outcomes measurement is nonetheless useful in assessing provider or institutional quality of care for high volume and relatively homogeneous procedures where technical skill is a factor. These comparisons must be made with caution, given the inevitable influence of unrecognized confounding through selection biases inherent in routine practice. The use of well-validated risk adjustment algorithms is imperative to improve the chances that differences in outcomes arise from the technical quality of care provided, rather than from differences in prognostic characteristics of patients themselves. Observational outcomes studies can also be undertaken cautiously to illustrate unanticipated harm from interventions, test the external validity of randomized trial results, generate hypotheses about interventions that may be worth testing with formal experimental designs, and, very rarely, provide an acceptable level of evidence for adopting a particular intervention.

To reduce general inconsistencies in the uptake of evidence into practice, and to redress instances where process or outcomes of clinical care are measured and found wanting, several proven strategies are available. First, while new evidence published in journals or distilled into educational materials and practice guidelines does change practice through passive diffusion, evidence is most likely to have an impact if actively disseminated and made relevant and salient locally to practitioners. Strategies to achieve this end include:

- reminder systems
- concurrent audit and feedback
- local outreach through academic detailing
- patient-mediated interventions
- local involvement of an educationally influential practitioner, and
- a local needs assessment with a consensus among providers on the issues as well as the barriers and facilitators to positive change.

In conclusion, the practitioner of evidence-based cardiovascular medicine and surgery is increasingly challenged to stay abreast of his or her field and to maintain technical competence in performing ever more exacting procedures. Information systems in practice can and will be re-engineered to be more conducive to evidence-based clinical decision making. However, it will also remain important to assess practice patterns on a systematic basis, to share that information with patients and providers, and wherever necessary, take steps to improve physician performance with a view to optimizing the quality, accessibility, and efficiency of cardiovascular care.

References

1. Payne N, Saul C. Variations in use of cardiology services in a health authority: comparison of coronary artery revascularisation rates with prevalence of angina and coronary mortality. *BMJ* 1997;**314**:257–61.
2. Alter DA, Naylor CD, Austin P, Tu JV. Effects of socioeconomic status on access to invasive cardiac procedures and on mortality after acute myocardial infarction. *N Engl J Med* 1999;**341**:1359–67.
3. Anderson GM, Grumbach K, Luft HS, Roos LL, Mustard C, Brook R. Use of coronary artery bypass surgery in the United States and Canada. Influence of age and income. *JAMA* 1993;**269**:1661–66.
4. Krieger J, Collier C, Song L, Martin D. Linking community-based blood pressure measurement to clinical care: a randomized controlled trial of outreach and tracking by community health workers. *Am J Public Health* 1999;**89**:856–61.
5. Tu JV, Naylor CD, Austin P. Temporal changes in the outcomes of acute myocardial infarction in Ontario, 1992–1996. *Can Med Ass J* 1999;**161**:1257–61.
6. Jha P, Deboer D, Sykora K, Naylor CD. Characteristics and mortality outcomes of thrombolysis trial participants and non-participants: a population-based comparison. *J Am Coll Cardiol* 1996;**27**:1335–42.
7. Jollis JG, Ancukiewicz M, DeLong ER, Pryor DB, Muhlbaier LH, Mark DB. Discordance of databases designed for claims payment versus clinical information systems. Implications for outcomes research. *Ann Intern Med* 1993;**119**:844–50.
8. Hannan EL, Kilburn H, Jr, Lindsey ML, Lewis R. Clinical versus administrative data bases for CABG surgery. Does it matter? *Med Care* 1992;**30**:892–907.
9. Fisher ES, Whaley FS, Krushat WM *et al.* The accuracy of Medicare's hospital claims data: progress has been made, but problems remain. *Am J Public Health* 1992;**82**:243–8.
10. Dixon J, Sanderson C, Elliott P, Walls P, Jones J, Petticrew M. Assessment of the reproducibility of clinical coding in routinely collected hospital activity data: a study in two hospitals. *J Public Health Med* 1998;**20**:63–9.
11. Green J, Wintfeld N. How accurate are hospital discharge data for evaluating effectiveness of care? *Med Care* 1993;**31**: 719–31.
12. Krumholz HM, Chen J, Murillo JE, Cohen DJ, Radford MJ. Admission to hospitals with on-site cardiac catheterization facilities :impact on long-term costs and outcomes. *Circulation* 1998;**98**:2010–16.
13. Every NR, Larson EB, Litwin PE *et al.* The association between on-site cardiac catheterization facilities and the use of coronary angiography after acute myocardial infarction. Myocardial Infarction Triage and Intervention Project Investigators. *N Engl J Med* 1993;**329**:546–51.
14. Di Salvo TT, Paul SD, Lloyd-Jones D *et al.* Care of acute myocardial infarction by noninvasive and invasive cardiologists: procedure use, cost and outcome. *J Am Coll Cardiol* 1996;**27**:262–9.
15. Rochon PA, Anderson GM, Tu JV *et al.* Age- and gender-related use of low-dose drug therapy: the need to manufacture low-dose therapy and evaluate the minimum effective dose. *J Am Geriatr Soc* 1999;**47**:954–9.
16. Krumholz HM, Radford MJ, Wang Y, Chen J, Marciniak TA. Early beta-blocker therapy for acute myocardial infarction in elderly patients. *Ann Intern Med* 1999;**131**:648–54.
17. Evans RG. Introduction. In: Evans RG, Barer ML, Marmor TR, eds. *Why are some people healthy and others not? The determinants of health of populations.* New York: Aldine de Gruyter, 1994.
18. Fiebach NH, Viscoli CM, Horwitz RI. Differences between women and men in survival after myocardial infarction. Biology or methodology? *JAMA* 1990;**263**:1092–96.
19. Meehan TP, Radford MJ, Vaccarino LV *et al.* A collaborative project in Connecticut to improve the care of patients with acute myocardial infarction. *Conn Med* 1997;**61**:147–55.
20. White KL. Improved medical care statistics and the health services system. *Public Health Rep* 1967;**82**:847–54.
21. Outcomes and the management of health care. Health Services Research Group. *Can Med Ass J* 1992;**147**:1775–80.
22. Wennberg J, Gittelsohn. Small area variations in health care delivery. *Science* 1973;**182**:1102–8.
23. Wennberg J, Gittelsohn A. Variations in medical care among small areas. *Sci Am* 1982;**246**:120–34.
24. Wennberg JE, Barnes BA, Zubkoff M. Professional uncertainty and the problem of supplier-induced demand. *Soc Sci Med* 1982;**16**:811–24.
25. Wennberg J. Which rate is right? *N Engl J Med* 1986;**314**: 310–11.

26.Naylor CD. Grey zones of clinical practice: some limits to evidence-based medicine. *Lancet* 1995;**345**:840–2.
27.Diehr P, Cain KC, Kreuter W, Rosenkranz S. Can small-area analysis detect variation in surgery rates? The power of small-area variation analysis. *Med Care* 1992;**30**:484–502.
28.Diehr P, Cain K, Connell F, Volinn E. What is too much variation? The null hypothesis in small-area analysis. *Health Serv Res* 1990;**24**:741–71.
29.Petticrew M, McKee M, Jones J. Coronary artery surgery: are women discriminated against? *BMJ* 1993;**306**:1164–6.
30.Jaglal SB, Goel V, Naylor CD. Sex differences in the use of invasive coronary procedures in Ontario. *Can J Cardiol* 1994;**10**:239–44.
31.Ayanian JZ, Epstein AM. Differences in the use of procedures between women and men hospitalized for coronary heart disease. *N Engl J Med* 1991;**325**:221–5.
32.Krumholz HM, Douglas PS, Lauer MS, Pasternak RC. Selection of patients for coronary angiography and coronary revascularization early after myocardial infarction: is there evidence for a gender bias? *Ann Intern Med* 1992;**116**:785–90.
33.Gan SC, Beaver SK, Houck PM, MacLehose RF, Lawson HW, Chan L. Treatment of acute myocardial infarction and 30-day mortality among women and men. *N Engl J Med* 2000 **343**:8–15.
34.Weintraub WS, Kosinski AS, Wenger NK. Is there a bias against performing coronary revascularization in women? *Am J Cardiol* 1996;**78**:1154–60.
35.Chen E, Naylor CD. Variation in hospital length of stay for acute myocardial infarction in Ontario, Canada. *Med Care* 1994;**32**:420–35.
36.Quality of care: 1. What is quality and how can it be measured? Health Services Research Group. *Can Med Ass J* 1992;**146**:2153–8.
37.Quality of care: 2. Quality of care studies and their consequences. Health Services Research Group. *Can Med Ass J* 1992;**147**:163–7.
38.Naylor CD, Guyatt GH. Users' guides to the medical literature. XI. How to use an article about a clinical utilization review. Evidence-Based Medicine Working Group. *JAMA* 1996;**275**:1435–9.
39.Fibrinolytic Therapy Trialists' (FTT) Collaborative Group. Indications for fibrinolytic therapy in suspected acute myocardial infarction: collaborative overview of early mortality and major morbidity results from all randomised trials of more than 1000 patients. *Lancet* 1994;**343**:311–22.
40.The Heart and Stroke Foundation of Canada, the Canadian Cardiovascular Society and the Canadian Association of Emergency Physicians for the Emergency Cardiac Care Coalition. Recommendations for ensuring early thrombolytic therapy for acute myocardial infarction. *Can Med Ass J* 1996;**154**:483–7.
41.Rogers WJ, Bowlby LJ, Chandra NC *et al.* Treatment of myocardial infarction in the United States (1990 to 1993). Observations from the National Registry of Myocardial Infarction. *Circulation* 1994;**90**:2103–14.
42.Cox JL, Lee E, Langer A, Armstrong PW, Naylor CD. Time to treatment with thrombolytic therapy: determinants and effect on short-term nonfatal outcomes of acute myocardial infarction. Canadian GUSTO Investigators. Global Utilization of Streptokinase and + PA for Occluded Coronary Arteries. *Can Med Ass J* 1997;**156**:497–505.
43.Birkhead JS. Time delays in provision of thrombolytic treatment in six district hospitals. Joint Audit Committee of the British Cardiac Society and a Cardiology Committee of Royal College of Physicians of London. *BMJ* 1992;**305**:445–8.
44.GISSI–Avoidable Delay Study Group. Epidemiology of avoidable delay in the care of patients with acute myocardial infarction in Italy. A GISSI-generated study. *Arch Intern Med* 1995;**155**:1481–8.
45.Porter G, Doughty R, Gamble G, Sharpe N. Thrombolysis in acute myocardial infarction: reducing in hospital treatment delay. *N Z Med J* 1995;**108**:253–4.
46.Park RE, Fink A, Brook RH *et al.* Physician ratings of appropriate indications for six medical and surgical procedures. *Am J Public Health* 1986;**76**:766–72.
47.Brook RH, Chassin MR, Fink A, Solomon DH, Kosecoff J, Park RE. A method for the detailed assessment of the appropriateness of medical technologies. *Int J Technol Assess Health Care* 1986;**2**:53–63.
48.Park RE, Fink A, Brook RH *et al.* Physician ratings of appropriate indications for three procedures: theoretical indications vs indications used in practice. *Am J Public Health* 1989;**79**: 445–7.
49.Hamm CW, Reimers J, Ischinger T, Rupprecht HJ, Berger J, Bleifeld W. A randomized study of coronary angioplasty compared with bypass surgery in patients with symptomatic multivessel coronary disease. German Angioplasty Bypass Surgery Investigation (GABI). *N Engl J Med* 1994;**331**:1037–43.
50.King SB III, Lembo NJ, Weintraub WS *et al.* A randomized trial comparing coronary angioplasty with coronary bypass surgery. Emory Angioplasty versus Surgery Trial (EAST). *N Engl J Med* 1994;**331**:1044–50.
51.Coronary angioplasty versus coronary artery bypass surgery: the Randomized Intervention Treatment of Angina (RITA) trial. *Lancet* 1993;**341**:573–80.
52.Rodriguez A, Boullon F, Perez-Balino N, Paviotti C, Liprandi MI, Palacios IF. Argentine randomized trial of percutaneous transluminal coronary angioplasty versus coronary artery bypass surgery in multivessel disease (ERACI): in-hospital results and 1-year follow-up. ERACI Group. *J Am Coll Cardiol* 1993;**22**:1060–7.
53.Comparison of coronary bypass surgery with angioplasty in patients with multivessel disease. The Bypass Angioplasty Revascularization Investigation (BARI) Investigators. *N Engl J Med* 1996;**335**:217–25.
54.Hilborne LH, Leape LL, Bernstein SJ *et al.* The appropriateness of use of percutaneous transluminal coronary angioplasty in New York State. *JAMA* 1993;**269**:761–5.
55.Ayanian JZ, Landrum MB, Normand SL, Guadagnoli E, McNeil BJ. Rating the appropriateness of coronary angiography – do practicing physicians agree with an expert panel and with each other? *N Engl J Med* 1998;**338**:1896–1904.
56.Brook RH, Kosecoff JB, Park RE, Chassin MR, Winslow CM, Hampton JR. Diagnosis and treatment of coronary disease: comparison of doctors' attitudes in the USA and the UK. *Lancet* 1988;**1**:750–3.
57.McGlynn EA, Naylor CD, Anderson GM *et al.* Comparison of the appropriateness of coronary angiography and coronary

artery bypass graft surgery between Canada and New York State. *JAMA* 1994;**272**:934–40.

58.Chassin MR, Kosecoff J, Park RE *et al.* Does inappropriate use explain geographic variations in the use of health care services? A study of three procedures. *JAMA* 1987;**258**:2533–7.

59.Leape LL, Park RE, Solomon DH, Chassin MR, Kosecoff J, Brook RH. Does inappropriate use explain small-area variations in the use of health care services? *JAMA* 1990;**263**: 669–72.

60.Wennberg JE. The paradox of appropriate care. *JAMA* 1987;**258**:2568–9.

61.Tu JV, Naylor CD, Kumar D, DeBuono BA, McNeil BJ, Hannan EL. Coronary artery bypass graft surgery in Ontario and New York State: which rate is right? Steering Committee of the Cardiac Care Network of Ontario. *Ann Intern Med* 1997;**126**:13–19.

62.Naylor CD, Sykora K, Jaglal SB, Jefferson S. Waiting for coronary artery bypass surgery: population-based study of 8517 consecutive patients in Ontario, Canada. The Steering Committee of the Adult Cardiac Care Network of Ontario. *Lancet* 1995;**346**:1605–9.

63.Hux JE, Naylor CD. Are the marginal returns of coronary artery surgery smaller in high-rate areas? The Steering Committee of the Provincial Adult Cardiac Care Network of Ontario. *Lancet* 1996;**348**:1202–7.

64.Yusuf S, Zucker D, Peduzzi P *et al.* Effect of coronary artery bypass graft surgery on survival: overview of 10-year results from randomised trials by the Coronary Artery Bypass Graft Surgery Trialists Collaboration. *Lancet* 1994;**344**:563–70.

65.Goldberg KC, Hartz AJ, Jacobsen SJ, Krakauer H, Rimm AA. Racial and community factors influencing coronary artery bypass graft surgery rates for all 1986 Medicare patients. *JAMA* 1992;**267**:1473–7.

66.Hadley J, Steinberg EP, Feder J. Comparison of uninsured and privately insured hospital patients. Condition on admission, resource use, and outcome. *JAMA* 1991;**265**:374–9.

67.Hannan EL, Kilburn H, Jr, O'Donnell JF, Lukacik G, Shields EP. Interracial access to selected cardiac procedures for patients hospitalized with coronary artery disease in New York State. *Med Care* 1991;**29**:430–41.

68.Laouri M, Kravitz RL, French WJ *et al.* Underuse of coronary revascularization procedures: application of a clinical method. *J Am Coll Cardiol* 1997;**29**:891–7.

69.Guadagnoli E, Landrum MB, Peterson EA, Gahart MT, Ryan TJ, McNeil BJ. Appropriateness of coronary angiography after myocardial infarction among Medicare beneficiaries. Managed care versus fee for service. *N Engl J Med* 2000;**343**:1460–6.

70.Hemingway H, Crook AM, Feder G *et al.* Underuse of coronary revascularization procedures in patients considered appropriate candidates for revascularization. *N Engl J Med* 2001;**344**:645–54.

71.Tu JV, Austin PC, Chan BT. Relationship between annual volume of patients treated by admitting physician and mortality after acute myocardial infarction. *JAMA* 2001;**285**:3116–22.

72.Alter DA, Naylor CD, Austin PC, Tu JV. Long-term MI outcomes at hospitals with or without on-site revascularization. *JAMA* 2001;**285**:2101–8.

73.Pilote L, Califf RM, Sapp S *et al.* Regional variation across the United States in the management of acute myocardial infarction. GUSTO-1 Investigators. Global Utilization of Streptokinase and Tissue Plasminogen Activator for Occluded Coronary Arteries. *N Engl J Med* 1995;**333**:565–72.

74.Yusuf S, Flather M, Pogue J *et al.* Variations between countries in invasive cardiac procedures and outcomes in patients with suspected unstable angina or myocardial infarction without initial ST elevation. OASIS (Organisation to Assess Strategies for Ischaemic Syndromes) Registry Investigators. *Lancet* 1998;**352**:507–14.

75.Tu JV, Austin P, Naylor CD, Iron K, Zhang H. Acute myocardial infarction outcomes in Ontario. In Naylor CD, Slaughter PM, eds. *Cardiovascular health and services in Ontario. An ICES Atlas.* Toronto: Institute for Clinical Evaluative Sciences, 1999.

76.Wen SW, Hernandez R, Naylor CD. Pitfalls in nonrandomized outcomes studies. The case of incidental appendectomy with open cholecystectomy. *JAMA* 1995;**274**:1687–91.

77.Rouleau JL, Moye LA, Pfeffer MA *et al.* A comparison of management patterns after acute myocardial infarction in Canada and the United States. The SAVE investigators. *N Engl J Med* 1993;**328**:779–84.

78.Mark DB, Naylor CD, Hlatky MA *et al.* Use of medical resources and quality of life after acute myocardial infarction in Canada and the United States. *N Engl J Med* 1994;**331**: 1130–5.

79.Pilote L, Racine N, Hlatky MA. Differences in the treatment of myocardial infarction in the United States and Canada. A comparison of two university hospitals. *Arch Intern Med* 1994;**154**:1090–6.

80.Fu Y, Chang WC, Mark D *et al.* Canadian-American differences in the management of acute coronary syndromes in the GUSTO IIb trial: one-year follow-up of patients without ST-segment elevation. Global Use of Strategies to Open Occluded Coronary Arteries (GUSTO) II Investigators. *Circulation* 2000;**102**:1375–81.

81.McClellan M, McNeil BJ, Newhouse JP. Does more intensive treatment of acute myocardial infarction in the elderly reduce mortality? Analysis using instrumental variables. *JAMA* 1994; **272**:859–66.

82.DeLong ER, Nelson CL, Wong JB *et al.* Using observational data to estimate prognosis: an example using a coronary artery disease registry. *Stat Med* 2001;**20**:2505–32.

83.Sackett DL. Bias in analytic research. *J Chronic Dis* 1979;**32**: 51–63.

84.Tu JV, Jaglal SB, Naylor CD. Multicenter validation of a risk index for mortality, intensive care unit stay, and overall hospital length of stay after cardiac surgery. Steering Committee of the Provincial Adult Cardiac Care Network of Ontario. *Circulation* 1995;**91**:677–84.

85.Krumholz HM, Chen J, Wang Y, Radford MJ, Chen YT, Marciniak TA. Comparing AMI mortality among hospitals in patients 65 years of age and older: evaluating methods of risk adjustment. *Circulation* 1999;**99**:2986–92.

86.Tu JV, Sykora K, Naylor CD. Assessing the outcomes of coronary artery bypass graft surgery: how many risk factors are enough? Steering Committee of the Cardiac Care Network of Ontario. *J Am Coll Cardiol* 1997;**30**:1317–23.

87.Rubin DB. Estimating causal effects from large data sets using propensity scores. *Ann Intern Med* 1997;**127**:757–63.

88.Rice N, Leyland A. Multilevel models: applications to health data. *J Health Serv Res Policy* 1996;**1**:154–64.

89.Diez-Roux AV, Link BG, Northridge ME. A multilevel analysis of income inequality and cardiovascular disease risk factors. *Soc Sci Med* 2000;**50**:673–87.

90.Duncan C, Jones K, Moon G. Context, composition and heterogeneity: using multilevel models in health research. *Soc Sci Med* 1998;**46**:97–117.

91.Standards, guidelines and clinical policies. Health Services Research Group. *Can Med Ass J* 1992;**146**:833–7.

92.Lomas J. Retailing research: increasing the role of evidence in clinical services for childbirth. *Milbank Q* 1993;**71**:439–75.

93.Grimshaw JM, Russell IT. Effect of clinical guidelines on medical practice: a systematic review of rigorous evaluations. *Lancet* 1993;**342**:1317–22.

94.Davis DA, Thomson MA, Oxman AD, Haynes RB. Changing physician performance. A systematic review of the effect of continuing medical education strategies. *JAMA* 1995;**274**: 700–5.

95.Oxman AD, Thomson MA, Davis DA, Haynes RB. No magic bullets: a systematic review of 102 trials of interventions to improve professional practice. *Can Med Ass J* 1995;**153**: 1423–31.

96.Barnett GO, Winickoff RN, Morgan MM, Zielstorff RD. A computer-based monitoring system for follow-up of elevated blood pressure. *Med Care* 1983;**21**:400–9.

97.Dickinson JC, Warshaw GA, Gehlbach SH, Bobula JA, Muhlbaier LH, Parkerson GR, Jr. Improving hypertension control: impact of computer feedback and physician education. *Med Care* 1981;**19**:843–54.

98.Pozen MW, D'Agostino RB, Selker HP, Sytkowski PA, Hood WB, Jr. A predictive instrument to improve coronary-care-unit admission practices in acute ischemic heart disease. A prospective multicenter clinical trial. *N Engl J Med* 1984; **310**:1273–8.

99.Pozen MW, D'Agostino RB, Mitchell JB *et al.* The usefulness of a predictive instrument to reduce inappropriate admissions to the coronary care unit. *Ann Intern Med* 1980;**92**:238–42.

100.Bradley EH, Holmboe ES, Mattera JA, Roumanis SA, Radford MJ, Krumholz HM. A qualitative study of increasing beta-blocker use after myocardial infarction: Why do some hospitals succeed? *JAMA* 2001;**285**:2604–11.

101.Tu JV, Austin P, Rochon PA, Zhang H. Secondary prevention after acute myocardial infarction, congestive heart failure and coronary artery bypass graft surgery in Ontario. In: Naylor CD, Slaughter PM, eds. *Cardiovascular health and services in Ontario: an ICES Atlas.* Toronto: Institute for Clinical Evaluative Sciences, 1999.

102.Decker B, MacInnes R. Assessing the importance of report cards rating patient satisfaction. *Health Syst Lead* 1997; **4**:16–18.

103.Hannan EL, Kilburn HJ, Racz M, Shields E, Chassin MR. Improving the outcomes of coronary artery bypass surgery in New York State. *JAMA* 1994;**271**:761–6.

104.Hannan EL, Siu AL, Kumar D, Kilburn H, Jr, Chassin MR. The decline in coronary artery bypass graft surgery mortality in New York State. The role of surgeon volume. *JAMA* 1995; **273**:209–13.

105.Green J, Wintfeld N. Report cards on cardiac surgeons. Assessing New York State's approach. *N Engl J Med* 1995; **332**:1229–32.

106.Schneider EC, Epstein AM. Influence of cardiac-surgery performance reports on referral practices and access to care. A survey of cardiovascular specialists. *N Engl J Med* 1996;**335**: 251–6.

107.Hannan EL, Siu AL, Kumar D, Racz M, Pryor DB, Chassin MR. Assessment of coronary artery bypass graft surgery performance in New York. Is there a bias against taking high-risk patients? *Med Care* 1997;**35**:49–56.

108.Schneider EC, Epstein AM. Use of public performance reports: a survey of patients undergoing cardiac surgery. *JAMA* 1998; **279**:1638–42.

109.Marshall MN, Shekelle PG, Leatherman S, Brook RH. The public release of performance data: what do we expect to gain? A review of the evidence. *JAMA* 2000;**283**:1866–74.

110.Ghali WA, Ash AS, Hall RE, Moskowitz MA. Statewide quality improvement initiatives and mortality after cardiac surgery. *JAMA* 1997;**277**:379–82.

111.O'Connor GT, Plume SK, Olmstead EM *et al.* A regional intervention to improve the hospital mortality associated with coronary artery bypass graft surgery. The Northern New England Cardiovascular Disease Study Group. *JAMA* 1996; **275**:841–6.

112.O'Connor GT, Plume SK, Olmstead EM *et al.* A regional prospective study of in-hospital mortality associated with coronary artery bypass grafting. The Northern New England Cardiovascular Disease Study Group. *JAMA* 1991;**266**: 803–9.

113.Malenka DJ, O'Connor GT. A regional collaborative effort for CQI in cardiovascular disease. Northern New England Cardiovascular Study Group. *Jt Comm J Qual Improv* 1995; **21**:627–33.

114.Tu JV, Naylor CD. Coronary artery bypass mortality rates in Ontario. A Canadian approach to quality assurance in cardiac surgery. Steering Committee of the Provincial Adult Cardiac Care Network of Ontario. *Circulation* 1996;**94**:2429–33.

115.Ivanov J, Weisel RD, David TE, Naylor CD. Fifteen-year trends in risk severity and operative mortality in elderly patients undergoing coronary artery bypass graft surgery. *Circulation* 1998;**97**:673–80.

116.Tu JV, Naylor CD. Coronary artery bypass mortality rates in Ontario. A Canadian approach to quality assurance in cardiac surgery. Steering Committee of the Provincial Adult Cardiac Care Network of Ontario. *Circulation* 1996;**94**:2429–33.

Index

Note: *v* denotes differential diagnosis or comparisons.

abdominojugular reflux test 18
ACE inhibitors *see* angiotensin converting enzyme (ACE) inhibitors
acetylsalicylic acid (ASA) *see* aspirin (acetylsalicylic acid)
ACP Journal Club 3–4, 43
active dissemination, clinical practice changes 82
acute coronary syndrome (ACS) *see* myocardial infarction (MI)
age, coronary artery disease risk and 24
alteplase *see* tissue-type plasminogen activator
AMI *see* myocardial infarction (MI), acute
amiodarone, atrial fibrillation, decision analysis 61, 65
angina
  clinical diagnosis 16, 24
  stable effort
    aspirin 67
    decision analysis 67
angiography *see* coronary angiography
angioplasty *see* percutaneous transluminal coronary angioplasty (PTCA)
angiotensin converting enzyme (ACE) inhibitors
  efficacy, evidence 34
  myocardial infarction, cost effectiveness 60–62, 64
ankle edema 16
Annals of Internal Medicine 44
antiarrhythmic agents, research evidence 7–8
aorta
  coarctation, clinical diagnosis 20
  dissection, clinical diagnosis 20
aortic stenosis
  clinical diagnosis 19, 20
  surgery, decision analysis 67
aortic valve
  replacement, decision analysis 61
  stenosis *see* aortic stenosis
apical impulse 17–18, 21
Aries 43
aspirin (acetylsalicylic acid)
  atrial fibrillation, decision analysis 56–58, 61, 65–66
  efficacy, evidence 34
atrial fibrillation (AF) 9
  clinical diagnosis 20–21
  decision analysis in management 56–58, 61, 65
audit
  criteria 74–75
    application and applicability 75, 76–77
    validity 75–18
  process-of-care 73–78
audit–feedback studies, clinical practice changes 82–83

β-2 adrenergic receptor, antagonists *see* β-blockers
β-blockers
  cost-effectiveness 54
  efficacy, evidence 34
balloon angioplasty *see* percutaneous transluminal coronary angioplasty (PTCA)
Bayes' theorem 26–27
bias *see* randomized controlled clinical trials (RCTs)
blood pressure (BP), measurement
  accuracy 19, 20
  factors affecting accuracy 20–21
British Medical Journal 44

CABG *see* coronary artery bypass grafting
Canada, appropriateness of service use 76, 77–78
Canada Institute for Scientific and Technical Information 41
captopril, decision analysis 61, 64
Captopril Prevention Project (CPP), randomized clinical trials 35
cardiac arrest, emergency medical services 61, 66
Cardiac Arrhythmia Suppression Trial (CAST) 52
Cardiac Care Network 84
cardiac failure, MEDLINE search strategies 41–43
cardiac transplantation, decision analysis 61, 66–67
cardiomegaly, clinical diagnosis 17–18
cardiovascular history 14
cardiovascular services
  appropriateness of use 75, 76, 77–78
  process-of-care studies 73–78
  resources 46, 47
CardLine 43
CAST (Cardiac Arrhythmia Suppression Trial) 52
CD Rom textbooks 44
central venous pressure (CVP), clinical assessment 18, 21
charges, *v* costs 48–49
CHD *see* coronary artery disease
chest pain *see also* angina
  coronary artery disease risk 24
  diagnostic usefulness 15–16, 21
chronic obstructive airways disease (COPD) 16–17
cigarette smoking, prediction of coronary artery disease 24
clinical assessment 14–22, 23–26
  critical appraisal of literature 15
  diagnosis 24
  prediction of patient outcome 26
  screening 23–26
  strategies to locate literature 14–15
  usefulness 15–22
clinical expertise 8–9
clinical guidelines 81–83
clinical practice 71–88
  assessing 71, 73–81
  changing 81–85
    audits 82–84
    incentives/disincentives 81–82
  data
    primary *v* secondary 72
    quality 72–73
  outcome studies *see* outcome studies
  process-of-care studies 73–78
    descriptive 73–74, 78–79
    use for policy inferences 77–78
    utilization reviews/clinical audits 73–78
  process–outcome relationships 71–81
clinical trials, randomized *see* randomized controlled clinical trials (RCTs)
clofibrate, randomized clinical trials 35
coarctation, aorta, clinical diagnosis 20
Cochrane Controlled Trials Registry (CCTR) 43
Cochrane Database of Systematic Reviews (CDSR) 43
Cochrane Library 43
Cochrane Review Methodology Database (CRMD) 43
cohort studies 72
confounding
  outcomes report cards 83
  outcome studies 80–81
  randomized clinical trials 37
Consumer Price Index 52
contrast media, low *v* high osmolality 60, 63
coronary angiography
  appropriateness of use 75, 76
  costs 47–48
  preoperative, decision analysis 66
coronary artery bypass grafting (CABG)
  appropriateness of use 75, 76, 77–78
  cost-effectiveness 53–54, 54
  economic aspects 47, 49–50
  outcomes measurement 83–84
  preoperative, decision analysis 61, 66
coronary artery disease (CAD; CHD)
  diagnosis
    clinical 16–17, 24
    incremental value of tests 23–33
    value of stress tests 23, 26–28, 30
  multivessel, PTCA *v* CABG 3
  non-invasive screening for severe CHD 24–26, 28–29, 30–31
  prediction of outcome 26, 29, 31
  prevention, decision analysis 63–64, 65–66
coronary care units (CCUs), in AMI 61, 66
Coronary Drug Project, intention to treat analysis 35
coronary heart disease (CHD) *see* coronary artery disease (CAD; CHD)
cost-benefit analysis 51

cost-effectiveness (CE)
analysis 51–55
decision analysis 58–60, 62
measuring effectiveness 52–53
new technologies 62–63
specific clinical products 63–66
treatment strategies 66–68
benchmarks 53
calculation 53
diagnostic tests 29–31, 54–55
patient selection and 53–54
ratio 53, 62
selected therapies 54
cost-minimization analysis 51, 53
costs 47–51
average 48
cost-effectiveness analysis 52
estimation 49–50
international perspectives 50–51
marginal 48, 49
staff 48
supply 47–48
v charges 48–49
counseling, physician, cost-effectiveness 54
Cox's linear proportional hazards model 29
cross-sectional studies 72
cross-subsidization 49

data *see* information
Database of Abstracts of Reviews of Effectiveness (DARE) 43
decision analysis 29–30, 56–70, 71
applications in cardiology 60–68
examples 56–60
modeling 6
new technologies 60, 62–63
specific clinical products 60–61, 63–66
treatment strategies 61–62, 66–68
decision node 56
decision tree 56, 57, 58–59, 59
evaluation 57–58, 59
folding back 58
diabetes mellitus, coronary artery disease prediction 24–25
diagnosis, MEDLINE search strategies 42
diagnostic tests 23–33 *see also* clinical assessment
approaches to assessing 26–29
clinical significance 29–31
cost-effectiveness 29–31, 54–55
diagnosis 26–28
incremental value 23–33
prognosis 29
screening 28–29
Digitalis Investigation Group (DIG) 38
discounting 52
dyspnea
diagnostic usefulness 16–17
paroxysmal nocturnal 16

ECG *see* electrocardiogram
economics *see also* costs
general concepts 47
health 46–55
international perspectives 50–51
effectiveness, measuring 52–53
electrocardiogram (ECG)
coronary artery disease 24–25, 26
decision analysis 68
mathematical correction 27
emergency medical services 61, 66
enalapril, cost-effectiveness 54
encainide, research evidence 7
etiology, MEDLINE search strategies 42
evidence based cardiology
about diagnosis, finding current 40–45
basic model 4
clinical expertise 8–9
clinical prediction tools 5
clinical state/circumstances 4–6
decision analytic modeling 6
definition 3–13
evolving model 4
example 4–5, 9, 10, 11
general approach 4–12
history 3
limitations 10–12
patient communication 8
patients' preferences/actions 6–7
randomized controlled trials 5, 7–8
research evidence 7–8
contradictions 8
hierarchy 7
limitations 7
value 7
variations 9
Evidence-Based Cardiovascular Medicine 43, 44
Evidence-Based Medicine 3–4, 43
exercise, cost-effectiveness 54, 55
exercise stress testing
incremental value 28–29, 30
mathematical correction 27

false negative results, randomized clinical trials 36
fibrinolytic (thrombolytic) therapy 75
decision analysis 61, 65
efficacy, evidence 34
flecainide, research evidence 7
Framingham Study, blood lipids 64

gender differences, coronary artery disease 24
geographic variations, clinical practice 73, 74
GISSI-1, subgroup analysis, inappropriate 36
gradings, definitions 2
guidelines
clinical 71
online 44
GUSTO-I trial, outcome studies 78, 79

health care
costs 46
outcomes *see* outcomes
quality *see* quality of care
Health Care Information Service 41
health economics 46–55
health services, research 71–73
heart failure, MEDLINE search strategies 41–43
heart rate, clinical assessment 20–21
hierarchical statistical modeling, outcome studies 80–81
hierarchy of evidence 7
high risk groups, value of identifying 31
history
cardiovascular 14
usefulness 15–17
hospital discharge abstracts 73
hyperlipidemia, prediction of coronary artery disease 24–25
hypoplastic left heart syndrome, decision analysis 67–68
hypotension, orthostatic 17
implantable cardioverter defibrillators (ICDs)
cost-effectiveness analysis 58–60
decision analysis 60, 62–63
incremental analysis 58
inflation 52
information, sources 40–45, 72
specialized 43
insurance databases 73
integrative reports 71
"intention to treat" analysis 35
internal jugular vein 18
Internet 44
intervention studies 72
ISIS-2, subgroup analysis drawbacks 36

JAMA 44
journals
keeping up to date 44
online 44
specialized 43
jugular venous pressure, "a" wave, clinical assessment 18

The Lancet 44
"law of diminishing returns" 47
learning opportunities 40
left ventricle (LV), dimension, enlargement, clinical diagnosis 17–18
left ventricular (LV) dysfunction, clinical diagnosis 17–18
levels of evidence, gradings 2
lifestyles
likelihood ratio (LR) 15
linear proportional hazards model 29
logistical regression analysis 28–29, 30
lovastatin, cost-effectiveness 54
Lp(a)
marginal costs 48, 49
Markov (state transition) models 58

Medical Matrix 40–41, 44
medical subject headings (MeSH) 41
MEDLINE 14, 40–43, 44
search strategies 42
meta-analyses *see* systematic overviews
mortality, cost-effectiveness analysis 52
murmurs, systolic, clinical assessment 18–19
myocardial infarction (MI)
acute (AMI)
clinical diagnosis 15–16, 16
coronary care unit (CCU) admission 61, 66
thrombolytic therapy *see* fibrinolytic (thrombolytic) therapy
decision analysis 68
previous history 24–25
myocardial ischemia *see also* angina
diagnosis 16–17

National Library of Medicine (NLM) 40–43
New England Journal of Medicine 44

observational studies
outcomes assessment 78–81
randomized clinical trials *v* 38
orthopnea 16–17
orthostatic hypotension 17
outcomes (endpoints)
anti-ischemic drugs
cost-effectiveness analysis 52–53
decision analysis 57, 59
categories 73
diagnostic test evaluation 23

economic aspects 47
quality of care studies 73, 78–79
studies *see* outcome studies
outcomes report cards 83–84
outcome studies 78–81
competing process factors 79
confounding 80–81
GUSTO-1 78, 79
hierarchical statistical modeling 80–81
non-randomized 80–81
process/outcome hypothesis 79
process–outcome relationships 78–81
propensity scores 80
quality of care 78–81, 79
risk-adjustment algorithms 80
selection bias 80
types 78–80
overhead, hospital 48
overviews, systematic *see* systematic overviews

panel methods 75
passive diffusion, clinical practice changes 81
patient communication 8
percutaneous transluminal coronary angioplasty (PTCA)
appropriateness of use 76–77
CABG *v* 75
economic aspects 49–50
physical activity, cost-effectiveness 54
physical examination 14
usefulness 17–21
PLAC study 64
post-test probability 26–27
post-test referral bias 27
pravastatin
cost-effectiveness 63–64
decision analysis 61
pretest probability 24, 26–27, 55
probability
decision analysis 57, 59
post-test 26–27
pretest 24, 26–27, 55
process of care 73
prognosis, MEDLINE search strategies 42
propensity scores, outcome studies 80
PTCA *see* percutaneous transluminal coronary angioplasty
"publication bias" 37
pulses, clinical assessment 20–21

quality-adjusted life years (QALYs) 52–53
quality-adjusted survival 57
quality of care
outcome studies 78–81, 79
process studies 73–78
quality of life, in cost-effectiveness analysis 52–53
quinidine, decision analysis 61, 65

radiofrequency (RF) ablation, cost-effectiveness 54
radionuclide angiography, exercise, incremental value 30
RAND group 75, 77–78
randomized controlled clinical trials (RCTs) 5, 7–8, 34–39, 71–72
compliance 35
confounding 37
false negative results 36
large scale 37–38
minimizing bias 34–37
data-dependent emphasis 35–36
intention to treat analysis 35
moderate 34–37
proper randomization 34–35
minimizing random errors 36–37
observational studies *v* 38
subgroup analysis, inappropriate 36
uncertainty principle 37–38
receiver operating characteristic (ROC) curves 28–29
recommendations, gradings 2
referral bias, post-test 27
reports, integrative 71
resources
cardiovascular care 46, 47
"law of diminishing returns" 47
risk-adjustment algorithms, outcome studies 80

SAVE (Survival and Ventricular Enlargement) trial, cost-effectiveness 64
Scandinavian Simvastatin Survival Study (4S), cost-effectiveness analysis 63
Scientific American Medicine (SAM) 44
screening, severe coronary artery disease 24–26, 28–29, 30–31
selection bias, outcome studies 80
sensitivity, analysis 57, 58, 60
significance, clinical, diagnostic tests 29–31
simvastatin
cost-effectiveness 63–64
decision analysis 60
single-intervention studies, clinical practice changes 82
smoking, prediction of coronary artery disease 24–25
societal perspective 52
state transition (Markov) models 58
streptokinase (SK), comparative trials 61, 65
stress tests, incremental value 23, 26–28, 30
stroke, prevention, decision analysis 56–58, 61, 65–66
sudden cardiac death, prevention by implantable cardioverter defibrillators 58–60, 62–63
survival
cost-effectiveness analysis 52–53
decision analysis 57
Survival and Ventricular Enlargement (SAVE) trial, cost-effectiveness 64
syncope
diagnostic evaluation 17
situational 17
systematic overviews (meta-analyses) 71
advantages 36
incomplete ascertainment 37
MEDLINE searching 41
publication bias 37
small scale 37
trial selection 37
unreliability 37

textbooks 43–44
online 44
thallium-201 imaging, incremental value 28–29, 30–31
third heart sound, clinical assessment 18
tissue-type plasminogen activator (tPA, alteplase)
comparative trials 61, 65
cost-effectiveness 54
treadmill exercise testing, incremental value 27–28, 30
treatment
cost-effectiveness 53–54
MEDLINE search strategies 42

uncertainty principle, randomized clinical trials 37–38
United Kingdom, appropriateness of service use 76
United States (USA), appropriateness of service use 76, 77–78
utilization review (clinical audit) 73–78

validity, audit criteria 75
vascular surgery, preoperative coronary revascularization 61, 66
vasovagal syndrome 17

warfarin, atrial fibrillation, decision analysis 53–58, 61, 65
Wolff–Parkinson–White (WPW) syndrome, treatment, decision analysis 60, 63